# Synopsis of General Pathology for Surgeons

**Biomedical Library**
Queen's University Belfast
Tel: 028 9097 2710
Email: biomed.info@qub.ac.uk

For due dates and renewals see
**'My Account'** at
http://qu-prism.qub.ac.uk/TalisPrism/

This book must be returned not later than
its due date, but is subject to
recall if in demand

Fines are imposed on overdue books

*For Linda, Titus, Alexander and Poppy*

# Synopsis of General Pathology for Surgeons

## D.W.K. Cotton

*PhD, MD, FRCPath*

*Reader in Pathology
Department of Pathology
University of Sheffield Medical School and
Honorary Consultant Pathologist to
The Royal Hallamshire Hospital, Sheffield*

*Examiner at the Royal College of Pathologists,
London*

*Member of the Court of Examiners of
the Royal College of Surgeons of England*

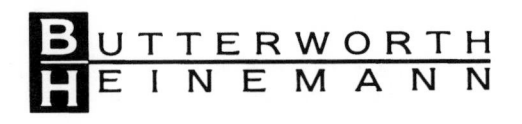

Butterworth-Heinemann
Linacre House, Jordan Hill, Oxford OX2 8DP
A division of Reed Educational and Professional Publishing Ltd

ℛ A member of the Reed Elsevier plc group

OXFORD   BOSTON   JOHANNESBURG
MELBOURNE   NEW DELHI   SINGAPORE

First published 1997

© Reed Educational and Professional Publishing Ltd 1997

**British Library Cataloguing in Publication Data**

Cotton, Dennis W.K.
  Synopsis of general pathology for surgeons
  1. Pathology, Surgical
  I. Title
  617'.07

ISBN  0 7506 3592 4

**Library of Congress Cataloguing in Publication Data**

Cotton, Dennis W.K.
  Synopsis of general pathology for surgeons/D.W.K. Cotton.
  p.   cm.
  Includes bibliographical references and index.
  ISBN  0 7506 3592 4
  1. Pathology.   2. Pathology, Surgical.   I. Title.
  [DNLM: 1. Pathology.   QZ 4 C8505s]
  RB111.C84
  616.07–dc21                                           97–938
                                                         CIP

Typeset by E & M Graphics, Midsomer Norton, Bath
Printed and bound in Great Britain by Biddles Ltd, Guildford and King's Lynn

# Contents

# Foreword

One's concept of a pathology textbook tends to conjure up visions
of a large dusty tome that lends itself ideally to the pressing of flowers.
Such an image is unfortunate because a sound understanding of
pathology is crucial to a safe and effective surgical practice. The
Court of Examiners of the Royal College of Surgeons of England
recognize all too well the vital importance of surgical pathology in
clinical practice and therefore a basic understanding of general
pathology will be examined both at Basic Surgical Training level
in the MRCS examination as well as at Higher Surgical Training level
in the Intercollegiate FRCS. Therefore to be presented with a
pathology textbook that addresses the subject of General Pathology in a
clear and didactic manner is indeed a windfall.

The aim of this book is to provide the surgical trainee as well as the
practising surgeon with a true synopsis of general pathology. This it
does with a high degree of clarity and commendable brevity. It does not
seek to be a reference book but to live up to its title and provide a
concise review of general pathology presenting the topic by disease
processes rather than by organ systems. The divide between systematic
and general pathology is dubious, if it exists at all, but this volume seeks
to address the topic in a way that is relevant to all systematic disease
processes. It is clearly laid out and contains most useful definitions of
terminology that can often prove confusing to a practising surgeon. The
content is comprehensive without being exhaustive and is ideal not only
for revision but also for general instruction in the principles and practice
of surgical pathology.

In preparing this volume, the author very much had in mind the
surgical trainee and the hurdles of postgraduate examinations. A
thorough understanding of the material presented in this book will
undoubtedly satisfy even the most demanding of postgraduate
examiners and indeed many of them may with benefit turn to its
pages themselves for inspiration and information. The author is ideally
placed to provide such insight and information, being an examiner

himself and I can therefore strongly recommend this volume to all aspiring surgeons as well as to all practising surgeons who wish to acquire a basic yet broad knowledge and understanding of surgical pathology.

**W.E.G. Thomas, MS, FRCS**
Consultant Surgeon and Clinical Director of Surgery,
The Royal Hallamshire Hospital, Sheffield

Court of Examiners and Surgical Skills Tutor of the Royal College of Surgeons of England, Intercollegiate Board of Examiners in General Surgery

# Preface

Having been an examiner for the Applied Basic Sciences section of the FRS for several years I have become aware that there is no suitable, brief textbook on basic pathology available. What I needed was a text from which I could select questions and which would also provide me with answers of suitable detail to allow me to know whether the candidates, myself and my colleagues were informed to the appropriate level. When faced with such a problem the traditional response is to write the book; this I have done.

The intention is to provide a synoptic text that is accurate and up-to-date and that will answer the questions which the candidates are likely to encounter. I was also concerned that the detail provided should be detailed enough but not too forbidding. Consequently the more detailed material is collected into tables for the enthusiast and recent references are supplied for even greater authority.

I have also tried to stay relevant to the surgical situation and avoid the recondite aspects of the pathology of the organ of Zuckerkandl whilst still providing current solid information regarding such matters as prions and antioncogenes.

I hope that readers will let me know of omissions with gentleness and that the book is useful to candidates during their encounters with the 'examiners from hell', as I believe we are sometimes fondly described.

# Acknowledgements

I should like to express my thanks to those numerous surgeon colleagues who asked questions that I could not answer and who thus prompted my further reading. It is a pleasure to acknowledge my debt to my publisher Dr Geoffrey Smaldon at Butterworth-Heinemann who thought that the project was a good idea and encouraged me to push it along; our telephone conversations have cheered me through many a difficult section!

The constant flow of ideas, argument, discussion, correction and downright awkwardness of my pathology colleagues in Sheffield is a constant source of stimulation and, in the particular case of this book, I would single out the kind help of Professor James Underwood and the harmonically advanced contributions of Dr Simon Cross.

# Introduction

Pathology is defined as the scientific study of disease. It is therefore a laboratory discipline. Modern pathology is divided into specialties including:

- histopathology (surgical pathology or diagnostic pathology);
- cytology (disaggregated cell preparations);
- morbid anatomy (autopsies);
- microbiology;
- chemical pathology;
- immunology;
- haematology.

These divisions have grown up for political reasons and there is no fundamental reason for separating them all. They are usually practised by separate specialists but in some places there are still general pathologists who may practise all or several of these disciplines.

The subject matter of histopathology is divided into two main branches:

- general pathology (preferred modern term is 'disease processes');
- systematic pathology.

General pathology is the study of the processes of pathology regardless of the organs in which they occur. The classifications of these vary from time to time as fashions and knowledge change but they generally include:

- cellular injury and cell death;
- disorders of growth, differentiation and morphogenesis;
- disorders of metabolism;
- haemodynamic disorders, ischaemia and shock;
- immunology and immunopathology;
- inflammation, repair and wound healing;
- carcinogenesis;
- neoplasia;
- ageing and individual death;
- infections.

The Royal College of Surgeons of England divides the subject matter up slightly differently:

- disorders of metabolism;
- cellular pathology;
- haematology and transfusion;
- microbiology and parasitology;
- disorders of circulation;
- causes of disease;
- inflammation and repair;
- disorders of growth;
- immunology and transplantation.

The differences are unimportant; the classifications are only there to prevent us forgetting things.

The classification of diseases is difficult for many reasons:

- scurvy is a metabolic disease caused by the inability of humans to synthesize vitamin C;
- scurvy is a dietary disease since it only occurs if the diet lacks vitamin C;
- tuberculosis is a bacterial disease;
- tuberculosis is more frequent in subjects with poor nutrition – it is therefore at least partly, a nutritional disease;
- glucose-6-phosphate dehydrogenase (G6PD) deficiency results in haemolytic disease and is therefore a genetic disease;
- people with 'normal' G6PD are more susceptible to malaria therefore this is the metabolic abnormality.

In a patient the disease usually presents together with the body's adaptive responses, i.e. infections present together with the signs of an inflammatory and immune response which are often the most distressing aspects of the disease and what the patient wants treated; suppressing these with steroids may worsen the patient's condition.

Systematic pathology is general pathology occurring in specific organs or systems or, in experimental pathology, other species.

It is the same pathology but it may be modified by the site in which it occurs, for instance:

- tumours in the general body may metastasize to brain;
- brain tumours do not metastasize into the rest of the body;
- in inflammation, skin becomes hotter (it approaches core temperature);
- an inflamed appendix is the same temperature as the other viscera;
- teratomas of the ovary are usually benign;
- teratomas of the testis are usually malignant;

- lack of vitamin C in the diet of man and guinea pigs causes scurvy;
- lack of vitamin C in the diet of rats causes no disease – they make their own;
- dogs and horses never suffer clavicular fractures – they don't have clavicles.

Why do surgeons need to know general pathology?

- As is your pathology so is your surgery (old surgical aphorism);
- Disease is treated better and more effectively by people who understand it;
- it is easier to remember things that you understand;
- innovation is more likely and much quicker if you know what is going on;
- you cannot understand the significance of lab reports if you do not understand pathology.

For all these reasons pathology is a requirement of surgical qualification.

Understanding pathology aids diagnosis:

- the problem with large breast tumours and thick melanomas is that they have already metastasized; you cannot treat metastasis with wider local excisions; radical mastectomies and dinner plate resections do not improve survival and carry their own extra morbidity;
- osteomata of the jaw and epidermal cysts occur in rare kindreds with polyposis coli (Gardner's syndrome);
- benign tumours rarely invade nerves; a parotid tumour with associated facial nerve palsy is likely to be malignant.

How should you study?

- attention spans are short – study in episodes that are within your attention span (little and often generally works best);
- learning works best visually – draw mind maps (see *Figures 6.1* and *9.1*) and pin them on the wall or door of the lavatory;
- eliminate distractions (some people are distracted by noise, some by silence);
- repetitions make truth (advertising aphorism) – recite your lists until they are perfect;
- think about the topic, digest it, summarize it, plan the next move;
- peer pressure works – form buzz groups to mock and degrade each other's ignorance (if you don't now, lawyers will later).

Don't kid yourself:

- looking at a page and saying 'I know this' is kidding yourself – shut

the book and write out a summary of the page (if you did know it, great, if you didn't then keep doing it until you do);
- watching 'soaps' on TV whilst learning is kidding yourself – you will learn the soap not pathology;
- kidding yourself is saying 'this won't come up' – oh yes it will!

Don't panic, it *can* be done; what many idiots have done before, you too can do.


## Bibliography

The best book is the book you read, others are just ornaments.

*Robbins Pathologic Basis of Disease*, 5th Ed, by Cotran R.S., Kumar V. and Robbins S.L., W.B. Saunders Co. (1994).
The best book on the subject, covers general and systematic pathology.

*General and Systematic Pathology*, 2nd Ed, edited by Underwood J.C.E., Churchill Livingstone (1996).
The most relevant undergraduate book, useful when you have forgotten some basic pathology (and who has not?).

*Cells, Tissues and Disease*, 1st Ed, by Majno G. and Joris, I., Blackwell Science (1996)
The most up-to-date and interesting book available on general pathology. Evaluates lots of recent experimental work.

**Journals:**
*Histopathology*
*Journal of Pathology*
*Journal of Clinical Pathology*
*British Medical Journal*
*Lancet*
All contain longer or shorter authoritative pathology reviews; worth scanning the reviews for the last year before the exam.

*Recent Advances in Histopathology*
*Progress in Pathology*
*Pathology Annual*
All contain longer, authoritative reviews; worth scanning the last couple of issues before the exam (many examiners do).

# Characteristics, classification and incidence of disease

Older styles of classification contained numerous categories that have now disappeared; as the causation of more diseases becomes clear, aetiological classifications are replacing older morphological ones.

## Definitions

Aetiology = the cause of a disease.
Pathogenesis = the means by which the cause produces the disease.
Disease = a process disturbing structure and/or function of the body either locally or systemically.

## Types of disease

- Congenital:
  (a) genetic
  (b) acquired
- Trauma
- Infections and infestations
- Inflammatory
- Metabolic
- Vascular
- Accumulations
- Immunological
- Iatrogenic
- Disorders of growth:
  (a) non-neoplastic
  (b) neoplastic:
    (i) benign
    (ii) malignant
- Ageing and death

## Definitions

Congenital = any disease present at birth.

Genetic = a disease caused by a mutated genome.

Acquired = a disease not inherent in the genome.

Trauma = diseases caused by external physical/chemical events (including poisons and radiation).

Infections and infestations = diseases caused by other living but small organisms.

Inflammatory = diseases where inflammation is the primary event and no other cause is known.

Metabolic = dynamic disturbances of metabolism.

Vascular = abnormalities of blood flow.

Accumulations = abnormal deposits of material in the cells or tissues.

Immunological = diseases where immunological processes are the primary event and no other cause is known.

Iatrogenic = caused by doctors.

Disorders of growth = diseases where a pathological alteration in size of the patient, an organ or a tissue is the main problem.

Neoplastic = a growth alteration in which there has been a mutation leading to an irreversible disorder of growth.

Benign neoplasm = not generally life-threatening.

Malignant neoplasm = generally life-threatening.

Ageing = slow, progressive decrease in vital function with time, associated with many other types of disease.

Death = the permanent disappearance of all signs of life.

## Examples

- Congenital:
  (a) genetic: Down's syndrome, cystic fibrosis, achondroplasia, thalassaemia;
- (b) acquired: thalidomide phocomelia, congenital syphilis, fetal drug dependency.
- Trauma: fractures, burns, poisoning, fat embolism, gunshot wounds.
- Infections: viral, fungal, bacterial, protozoan, helminthic.
- Infestations: (mostly arthropods) fleas, lice, scabies.
- Inflammatory: sarcoid, inflammatory bowel disease, psoriasis.
- Metabolic: gout, hypercalcaemia (secondary to tumours, diet, etc.).
- Vascular: myocardial ischaemia, embolism, shock.
- Accumulations: amyloidosis (secondary to neoplastic and inflammatory diseases), ochronosis, calcification (secondary to other diseases).
- Immunological: rheumatoid, lupus erythematosus, vitiligo.

- Iatrogenic: drug reactions, radiation scarring, surgical hernias.
- Disorders of growth:
  (a) non-neoplastic: dwarfism, acromegaly, reactive goitre;
  (b) neoplastic:
     (i) benign: naevocellular naevus (mole), uterine fibroids, mixed tumour of parotid;
     (ii) malignant: malignant melanoma, hepatocellular carcinoma, Hodgkin's lymphoma.
- Ageing: immunoparesis, cerebral atrophy, infertility (may all be secondary).
- Death:
  (a) cell death: necrosis, apoptosis;
  (b) somatic death: trauma, age-related, overwhelming disease.

## Problems with classification

- *Exceptions*: all systems of classification contain exceptions: some benign tumours can kill, e.g. pressure-effects of uterine fibroids can cause pulmonary emboli; basal cell carcinomas can erode into major vessels.
- *Overlap*: e.g. scurvy can be seen as a genetic deficiency, or a dietary deficiency, or a metabolic disease; berry aneurysms (Charcot–Bouchaud microaneurysms) are congenital vascular weaknesses or the results of hypertension (or perhaps neither).

Weller R.O. (1995) Subarachnoid haemorrhage and myths about saccular aneurysms. *J. Clin. Pathol.*, **48**, 1078–1081.

- *Ignorance*: 'spontaneous' inflammatory or immunological diseases presumably have a cause and may even be due to as yet unrecognized infections.
- *Alternatives*: many traditional categories of disease are disappearing as knowledge develops; metabolic diseases are easier to understand on the basis of aetiology (diabetes is caused by autoimmune loss of beta-cells in the pancreas; the mucopolysaccharidoses are better understood as lysosomal storage diseases associated with specific mutations in the DNA leading to deficiencies of the lysosomal enzymes responsible for the metabolism of various muco-polysaccharides).

## Systems of classification and numerical coding

- WHO produced *'International Classification of Disease'* (ICD) in 1948.

- College of American Pathologists produced '*Systematized Nomen-clature of Pathology*' (SNOP) in 1965.
- College of American Pathologists produced '*Systematized Nomen-clature of Medicine*' (SNOMED) in 1976 (currently widely used for computer storage and retrieval of clinical cases).

Classification and coding is discussed in:

Underwood J.C.E. (1987) *Introduction to Biopsy Interpretation and Surgical Pathology*, 2nd ed. Springer-Verlag, Berlin.

## Predisposition to diseases

- *Genetic*: mutations; some mutations lead directly to disease, e.g. a mutation in band q31-32 on chromosome 7 leads to a defective chloride channel protein cystic fibrosis transmembrane conductance regulator (CFTR), which results in a generalized abnormality in epithelial chloride transport.

    Other mutations only have an effect if the subject encounters an environmental trigger, e.g. mutations in the gene coding for erythro-cyte glucose-6-phosphate dehydrogenase result in haemolytic anaemia only when the patient is exposed to fava beans (favism) or certain drugs (antimalarials).
- *HLA type*: human leukocyte antigens (HLA) are the commonest and most varied genetic polymorphisms in humans, with two main classes:
    (a) class I: concerned with recognition by cytotoxic T-lymphocytes (in conjunction with viral antigens) on the surface of all nucleated cells;
    (b) class II: these antigens are present on the surface of those cells that normally interact with T-lymphocytes in the immune response, e.g. Langerhans cells in the epidermis.
    Specific immunophenotypes of both HLA classes are associated with a high risk for some diseases including infectious, autoimmune and neoplastic diseases
- *Sex*: some diseases show an absolute sex association, e.g. those carried on the Y-chromosome only occur in men and recessive genes carried on the X-chromosome only occur in women.

    Other associations are incomplete and statistical; autoimmune diseases are more common in women but also occur in men.
- *Race*: some racial associations with disease are related to geography rather than genetics and depend on cultural habits, diet or prevalence of parasites. Migrants then develop the disease patterns of their adopted homes.

Other race-related diseases are genetic and are due to relative restriction of a particular gene pool, migrants take their disease pattern with them.

# Epidemiology

The distribution of disease within populations in time and space is related to:

- genetic factors;
- nutritional factors;
- distribution of infectious agents;
- exposure to toxins, allergens, etc.;
- social factors (housing, behaviour, hygiene, etc.).

Knowledge depends upon:

- reliability of data (recognition of cases, registration of cases, reliability of reporting, compliance);
- methods of collection of data (local reporting, total registration, sampling, screening, death certification, autopsy rates);
- reliability of statistics (methodology, political manipulation);
- effects of screening, immunization, vector eradication, compliance, etc.

# Sampling methods for pathology

## Cytology

Cytology provides samples of disaggregated cells derived from tissues. There are two main sources of cytology:

- *exfoliative cytology* in which cells are scraped from tissue surfaces, such as cervical cytology and bronchial brushings;
- *fine-needle aspiration cytology* in which a fine-bore needle attached to a syringe is inserted into an organ and the plunger is withdrawn several times sucking up cells which are then spread onto a slide or placed in transport medium for transport to the laboratory.

### Advantages
- The technique is rapid.
- It does not require general anaesthetic.
- It can be performed as an office procedure.

## Disadvantages

- The architectural information in the lesion is lost.
- The sample is small compared to the tissue size but this is true for all sampling to various extents.

## Needle-core biopsy

A cutting needle (such as a Tru-cut) is used to obtain a core of tissue, which is then submitted for histology. The technique is often used for liver and prostate.

## Advantages

- The architecture is retained.
- The biopsy can be performed under radiological or ultrasound guidance.
- A general anaesthetic is rarely required.

## Disadvantages

- There is discomfort for the patient.
- It is more time consuming.
- The general problem of sample size.

## Frozen section

This is generally used as an intra-operative technique but can also be used to investigate substances such as fat that would be lost during routine processing for histology.

It was previously widely used in the surgery of breast lumps but has been relaced by the triple approach of clinical examination, mammography and cytology, since patients are distressed by not knowing the eventual extent of surgery when frozen section diagnosis is employed.

## Curettage

This is an office procedure, mainly employed by dermatologists who scrape off lesions from the skin and cauterize the base.

### Disadvantages

- It is not popular with pathologists, who rely on tissue architecture for many skin diagnoses (differentiation of keratoacanthoma from squamous carcinoma).
- Safety requires the dermatologist to be certain of the diagnosis before performing the procedure.

## Punch biopsy

This uses a sharp, hollow tube to take a core of tissue (mainly from skin).

It maintains tissue architecture but leaves a scar since the circular biopsy lesion is not easily sutured.

## Routine histology

Histology provides the best samples and the best results. It is used diagnostically and the surgeon can generally see what they are sampling and can describe the gross pathology on the request form.

### Advantages

- With large resections the material can be sent fresh and uncut to the laboratory.
- It can be adequately and accurately fixed (in $10 \times$ volume of fixative).
- Samples can be taken for special techniques (such as electron microscopy and immunofluorescence) if they are required.

# Incidence, prevalence, remission rate, mortality rate

## Definitions

- Incidence = the number of new cases occurring in a group of defined size during a defined period; this is a *rate* and specific values depend on the values given to the group size and the period length.
- Prevalence = the number of cases present in a defined group at a defined time; this is also a rate and it depends on the size of the denominator group.
- Remission rate = the number of cases in a defined group that recover.
- Mortality rate = the number of cases in a defined group that die.

## Data

- All such population statistics depend upon the reliability of the data and this may vary greatly from disease to disease, from time to time and from place to place.
- Many studies use death certification data, but most death certificates, even in developed countries, are written without the benefit of autopsy information and are very unreliable.

Start R.D. and Cotton D.W.K. (1996) The current status of the autopsy. *Progress in Pathology*, **3**, 179–188.

- Using such data, correlations with other data may be exposed (diet, geography, behaviour, etc.); this may not be taken as indicating a causative relationship, it is only a correlation (there is a correlation between benign breast disease and breast cancer, but this is because both are produced by the same factors, the one does not cause the other).
- In comparing data from two different sources it may be necessary to correct for differences in age or sex distribution or for some other factor; these rates are called *standardized* rates

# 2

# Mechanisms and responses to cellular injury and death

- Cells are the *anatomic* units of tissues or organs.
- The *functional* units may be unicellular or multicellular (glands, liver acini, nuclei in the brain).
- Cells consist of compartmentalized biochemical functions, many of which are separated by membranes.
- Cellular organelles are also defined by membranes.
- Membranes are active metabolic structures whose functions include *isolation* of metabolic events and *control of flow* of metabolites.
- Cell damage is commonly, but not exclusively, due to disturbed membrane function.
- Cell damage may be reversible (sublethal) or lethal.
- The degree to which a tissue can replace damaged cells varies:
  (a) labile cells = good ability to regenerate, e.g. *epithelia*;
  (b) stable cells = low rate of division under normal circumstances but retain capacity to divide, e.g. *hepatocytes* and *renal tubular cells*;
  (c) permanent cells = no capacity for division, e.g. *nerve cells* and *striated muscle*.
- Postmitotic or terminally differentiated cells cannot divide and when lost are replaced by the division of stem cells; those best studied are intestinal crypt cells.

Wright N.A. (1984) Cell proliferation in health and disease. *Recent Adv. Histopathol.*, **12**, 17–33.

## Causes of cell injury

- Physical: mechanical, heat, cold, ionizing radiation.
- Chemical: poisons, drugs, hypoxia, nutritional derangements.
- Biological: infectious organisms, prions.
- Immunological: autoimmune disease, complement.
- Genetic: inborn errors of metabolism.

Prusiner S.R. (1995) The prion diseases. *Sci. Am.*, **Jan**, 30–37.

# Consequences of injury

These depend upon:

- the nature of the injurious agent;
- the duration of the insult;
- the extent of the injury (what proportion and type of the cells are lost);
- the severity of the injury (degree of burns, degree of crush, shock waves in high velocity missile injury, strength of acids, dose of drugs);
- susceptibility of tissues (effects of oxygen depletion more rapid in brain than liver);
- degree of damage to repair mechanisms (disruption of blood and nerve supply, acquired immuno deficiency syndrome (AIDS), inability to absorb nutrients or to respire).

# Histological and electron microscopical appearance of damaged cells

- Hydropic change: swollen pale cells due to damage to calcium export mechanisms allowing calcium in, which is followed by water.
- Fatty change: accumulation of fat in the cell due to various processes such as uncoupling of lipid and protein metabolism (common in liver).
- Eosinophilia: disappearance of mRNA from cytoplasm removes some haematoxylin staining leaving eosin staining more prominent.
- Swollen mitochondria: damage to calcium export allowing calcium in, which is followed by water.
- Smooth endoplasmic reticulum (ER): dilatation.
- Rough ER: loss of ribosomes.
- Nuclear changes: clumping of chromatin (pyknosis), progressive breakdown of chromatin (karyorrhexis, karyolysis).

# Mechanisms of cell damage

- Four processes mediate the majority of cell injury whatever the initiating factor:
  - (a) oxygen supply and oxygen free radicals;
  - (b) disturbances in calcium homeostasis;
  - (c) depletion of ATP;
  - (d) membrane damage.

- Lack of oxygen causes the cell to switch from aerobic mitochondrial metabolism to anaerobic glycolysis which uses glycogen to produce ATP.
- Glycolysis is less efficient than aerobic metabolism so glycogen and ATP stores fall.
- Glycolysis is also incomplete metabolism of sugars so lactic acid accumulates and pH falls; this results in nuclear chromatin clumping.
- Control of water influx into the cell is ATP-dependent so cell swelling occurs.
- Adherence of ribosomes to ER is also ATP-dependent and these separate during ischaemia.
- Similar effects occur in the mitochondria.
- Calcium influx occurs into the cell and into mitochondria.
- This is made worse at this stage if the ischaemia is reversed (reperfusion injury) since some cell damage is oxygen-dependent (apoptosis).
- If ischaemia continues, lysosomal leakage occurs and hydrolytic enzymes attack cell constituents.
- Leakage of specific cell constituents provides a clinical test for cell damage, e.g. cardiac isoenzymes in the blood in myocardial infarction.
- Cell death occurs when these changes become irreversible.
- The precise cause of cell death is not known but membrane damage, cytoskeletal disorganization, loss of phospholipids, accumulation of lipid metabolites and loss of intracellular amino acids all seem to contribute.

## Free radical damage

- Major cause of membrane damage.
- Final common pathway in many different forms of injury.
- Free radicals have a single, unpaired electron in their outer orbit which makes them highly chemically reactive with most biological molecules.
- They react with cell and organelle membranes by lipid peroxidation; they can cross-link and otherwise damage proteins and DNA.
- They are autocatalytic so a small initial amount does much damage.
- The cell contains numerous chemicals and processes to inactivate free radicals and these need oxygen to be regenerated.
- Free radicals are also produced by exogenous causes such as ultra-violet (UV) or X-irradiation and by many drugs and chemicals (e.g nitric oxide or iron).

- Metabolic 'detoxification' of some drugs and chemicals generates free radicals.
- They are produced in many oxidative processes in the cell.
- The commonest metabolic oxidation free radicals are superoxide, hydrogen peroxide and hydroxyl ions and nitric oxide.
- They are very unstable compounds and decay spontaneously. There are enzymes such as superoxide dismutase and glutathione peroxidase that destroy them and some antioxidant chemicals block their formation or absorb them (free radical sinks or scavengers), e.g. cysteine, glutathione and some proteins.
- Regeneration of sinks or scavengers is ATP-dependent.

Springall D.R. (1995) Nitric oxide – friend and foe. *J. Pathol.*, **175**, 165–166.

# Reperfusion injury

- Under normal circumstances and directly following ischaemic injury the tissue concentrations of free radicals are very low.
- When perfusion is re-established the concentration of free radicals increases markedly.
- This leads to the paradox that re-establishing circulation and removing ischaemia leads to further tissue damage.
- These studies have been carried out on experimental animals by occluding vessels for various lengths of time and  killing the animals after the signs of tissue damage have had time to develop.
- Most tissue damage under these circumstances is due to polymorphs which enter the tissue following restoration of blood flow.
- If blood flow is not established, the affected tissue still dies but other mechanisms are responsible.
- The process is only paradoxical because unexpected and, in that sense,  is an artefact of the experimental system (though it may occur in myocardial infarction (MI) following thrombolytic therapy).

# Cell death

## Definitions

Necrosis = confluent cell death.
Apoptosis = single cell death, active process requiring energy and protein production.
Satellite necrosis = apoptosis associated with one or more lymphocytes.
Programmed cell death = predestined, energy-dependent cell death;

does not occur in adult human and is not the same as apoptosis; found in lower animals.

## Apoptosis
### *Morphology*

- There is single cell death which can occur in most tissues.
- It results in apoptotic bodies, sometimes containing nuclear debris.
- Apoptotic bodies are taken up and recycled by other cells of the same tissue (uncommonly by polymorphs or macrophages).
- Early signs include surface blebbing of the cell, margination of chromatin followed by cell contraction and break-up into one or more apoptotic bodies.
- Nuclear changes include chromatin clumping and breakdown appearance depends on the type of cell:
  - (a) epidermal cells with large amounts of cytoskeleton will be pink and amorphous and may be extruded into the dermis and taken up by macrophages;
  - (b) cells with a small amount of cytoplasm may be much smaller and darker because of dominance by nuclear remnants.
- Different names are used in different tissues: Civatte (or colloid) bodies in lichen planus; Kamino bodies in melanocytic lesions; Councilman bodies in acute viral hepatitis.

### *Mechanisms*

- Apoptosis probably evolved from genes used for remodelling during development and then became linked to processes for cell recognition and then became a means of killing a cell that was parasitized by a virus, but the pathway can also be activated by drugs, toxins and physical agents such as radiation.
- Apoptosis is seen in growing tissues and it may be responsible for the slow growth of tumours, such as basal cell carcinoma, where the mitotic rate is high.
- Endonucleases are produced as an early biochemical step and these act by cleaving DNA into short, double-stranded fragments: an irreversible step.
- In contrast to necrosis, calcium influx into the cell is an active process in apoptosis.
- Experimentally apoptosis can be inhibited by blocking RNA or protein synthesis.

**Table 2.1 Factors known to affect apoptosis**

| Factors involved in apoptosis | Effects and modes of action |
| --- | --- |
| Bcl-2 (B-cell lymphoma/leukaemia-2 gene) | One of several 'survival genes' that prevent apoptosis until a 'trigger gene' is activated. Gene product is membrane located |
| p53 | Tumour suppressor 'trigger' gene. Located on chromosome 17p and mutation and heterozygosity are associated with many cancers. Associated with apoptosis in cells with damaged DNA. Suggested that p53 may stall cells in $G_1$ to allow DNA repair and to trigger apoptosis if this fails |
| c-myc | Cellular oncogene which binds with protein max and binds to specific DNA sites in the vicinity of genes concerned with cellular growth such as PDGF |
| Glucocorticoids | Strongly stimulate apoptosis. They stimulate the production of calmodulin mRNA (a calcium binding protein) and may influence calcium flux into the cell which is an early step in apoptosis |
| APO-1 or Fas | Membrane antigen member of the superfamily of tumour necrosis factor receptor/nerve growth factor receptor cell surface proteins; antibodies to this antigen strongly stimulate apoptosis |
| T-cell antigen receptor in thymocytes | Stimulation of immature thymocytes results in apoptosis, stimulation of mature thymocytes results in cell activation. May protect against an immature and incomplete response |

PDGF, platelet-derived growth factor.

Chen S.-C., Curran T. and Morgan J.I. (1995) Apoptosis in the nervous system: new revelations. *J. Clin. Pathol.*, **48**, 7–12.
Cotton D.W.K. (1995) Death; the cell. *Prog. Pathol.*, **2**, 1–11.

## Macroscopic features of necrosis

Necrosis is death of tissue within the living organism. The type depends on the nature of the tissue and the causative agent:

- *coagulative*: presumably due to 'coagulation' of globular (enzymatic) proteins leaving cell outlines intact (characteristic of hypoxic death in all tissues except brain);
- *liquefactive* (colliquative): mostly seen in bacterial infections due to the attraction of polymorphs and their degradative enzymes; also occurs in brain hypoxia without infection;

- *caseous*: form of coagulative necrosis typical of tuberculosis;
- *gangrene*: not really a distinct form of necrosis but a clinical term applied to dead tissue in the body. When ischaemic, as in diabetes, it is 'dry', when bacterial, as in Clostridia infections, it is 'wet';
- *fibrinoid*: necrosis of smooth muscles in arterial walls in malignant hypertension; commonly there is no necrosis and the term is a misnomer;
- *fat*: either mechanical damage to fat (e.g. trauma to the breast) or enzymatic due to lipases (e.g. pancreatic inflammation).

## Tissue response to cell death

- Inflammation: a stereotypical response to any tissue damage which often evolves into a specific reaction pattern (see Chapter 4).
- Regeneration: return to normal tissue following injury. This depends on preservation of reticulin framework and labile cells, also to some extent on complexity of architecture (renal tubules may regenerate, glomeruli do not).
- Repair: replacement of original tissue by scar (e.g. fibrous scar in myocardium following myocardial infarction).

## Histological timing of tissue death

On a histology slide all the tissue is dead; what the pathologist looks for are features which show that tissue was dead before the specimen was taken for histology (*Table 2.2*).

**Table 2.2  Timing of pathological changes following myocardial infarction (Lee, 1995)**

| Time after death | Histological and EM features |
| --- | --- |
| 20–40 min | Earliest EM changes, swelling of mitochondria and ER |
| 1–3 h | Muscle fibres appear wavy |
| Up to 8 h | No histological changes but staining with tetrazolium dye positive at 2–3 h |
| 24–48 h | Oedema, acute inflammatory cell infiltrate, myocyte necrosis |
| 3–4 days | Obvious necrosis and inflammation, early granulation tissue |
| 1–3 weeks | Granulation tissue with progressive fibrosis |
| 3–6 weeks | Dense fibrosis, loss of inflammation and granulation tissue |

EM, electron microscope; ER, endoplasmic retilinlum.

Lee J.A. (1995) The pathology of cardiac ischaemia: cellular and molecular aspects. *J. Pathol.*, **175**, 167–174.

# Disorders of growth, morphogenesis and differentiation

- In the normal adult, tissue or organ size is constant and is a balance between cell size, cell loss, cell replacement and the amount of stroma.
- In tissues constructed from labile cells all of these processes may be modified by a wide range of influences.
- Growth, morphogenesis and differentiation are similar processes in the developing embryo and fetus and in the adult but the situations in which they occur and their end-results are different.
- During development the adult size and shape is achieved by selective variations in the elements of growth.
- Following injury with loss of tissue these processes are activated and accessory ones are called into play.
- During development, specific tissues arise from uncommitted cells by a process of differentiation.
- Following damage with tissue loss, uncommitted, or partially committed, cells may differentiate to replace lost cells.
- Regeneration takes place by division and differentiation of uncommitted *stem* or *reserve* cells.

## Types of physiological growth

Physiological growth takes place by several mechanisms:
- increase in number of cells (multiplication);
- increase in size of cells (auxetic);
- increase in intercellular tissue (accretionary);
- combined patterns.

## Cell cycle

- Somatic cells increase in numbers by mitosis; between mitoses the cells are in various stages of synthesis and rest, the whole process being known as the *cell cycle*.

- The cell cycle consists of four phases: M, $G_1$, S and $G_2$ with a further phase outside of the cycle called $G_0$.
- During the M phase *mitosis* occurs.
- During the S phase DNA is *synthesized*.
- $G_1$ and $G_2$ are *gap* phases.
- $G_0$ is a phase outside the cycle and some cells enter this permanently, lose the ability to mitose and are then *terminally differentiated* cells.
- The entry of cells into the various phases of the cycle is controlled by a group of proteins called *cyclins*.
- Some oncogenes are involved in the control of the cell cycle (*Bcl-1*, the anti-oncogene *Rb* and possibly *p53*).
- Various cancer therapeutic agents attack specific parts of the cell cycle.

## Stem (reserve) cells

- In a terminally differentiated cell population there are resting cells which can divide and differentiate to replace lost cells.
- Such cells are not differentiated but are determined, i.e. they will only develop into one sort of cell unless they are diverted by some pathological stimulus (metaplasia).
- Myocardium and nerve cells have no stem cells to replace losses.

Hall P.A. (1992) Differentiation, stem cells and tumour histogenesis. *Recent Adv. Histopathol.*, **15**, 1–15.

## Factors affecting growth

### Normal growth

Normal growth requires a number of factors whose absence results in limited or abnormal growth, these include:

- appropriate genetic constitution;
- adequate vascularization;
- adequate nutrition (proteins, vitamins, etc.);
- adequate oxygen;
- normal innervation;
- hormones;
- local growth factors (GFs).

## Pathology

- *Genetic disorders include*:
  - (a) achondroplasia, disproportionate growth retardation, the growth plates in the long bones where premature deposition of horizontal struts of bone seal the plate preventing further growth; the cause is unknown. Eighty per cent are new heterozygous mutations; homozygous forms occur with two achondroplasic parents;
  - (b) Beckwith–Weidemann syndrome is due to duplication of the short arm of chromosome 11 where the genes for insulin and somatomedin insulin-like growth factor (IGF)-2 reside, resulting in excessive growth.
- *Vascularization*: maldevelopment of a vessel can lead to non-development of the organ in its distribution.
- *Nutrition*: general catabolic states (such as may occur postsurgery) may induce severe weight loss with poor wound healing; general protein and protein calorie deficiencies result in kwashiorkor or marasmus.
- *Oxygen*: babies born at altitudes of 15 000 feet have 16% lower birthweight due to reduced oxygen pressure.
- *Nerve supply*: interrupted nerve supply leads to disuse atrophy but there is also a direct effect.
- *Hormones*:
  - (a) general body size is controlled by the pituitary growth hormone (GH), release of which is stimulated by hypothalamic growth hormone-releasing factor (GHRF) and inhibited by somatostatin;
  - (b) GH stimulates the release of somatomedins IGF-1 and IGF-2 from the liver; these act on target tissues such as muscle and bone;
  - (c) reduced GH in childhood leads to proportionate dwarfism; reduced GH receptors leads to Laron dwarfism; increased GH from pituitary adenoma in childhood produces gigantism and, after puberty, acromegaly because the epiphyses in long bones have fused.
- *Local growth factors*:
  - (a) in healing skin, platelets release platelet-derived growth factor (PDGF) and transforming growth factor beta (TGF-$\beta$) which attract inflammatory cells;
  - (b) in the epidermis PDGF and epidermal growth factor (EGF) act together to stimulate basal cell division; PDGF moves cells from $G_0$ to $G_1$ and EGF and the IGFs guide the cells from $G_1$ to DNA synthesis; in the epidermis EGF is derived from epidermal cells (autocrine and paracrine) and the IGFs from the circulation (endocrine) as well as from epidermal and dermal cells (autocrine and paracrine);

**Table 3.1 Some common cytokines and their actions**

| Cytokine | Features |
| --- | --- |
| EGF (epidermal growth factor) | Binds to EGF transmembrane receptor on most mammalian cells (most numerous on epithelial cells) and causes relative de-differentiation and proliferation |
| FGF (fibroblast growth factor) | Exists in two forms, acidic and basic (10 times more active); mitogenic for many mesenchymal cells and causes proliferation of capillaries |
| MDGF (macrophage-derived growth factor) | Secretion from macrophages stimulated by fibronectin and Gram-negative endotoxins; stimulates proliferation of quiescent fibroblasts, endothelial cells and smooth muscle cells |
| PDGF (platelet-derived growth factor) | Stored in α-granules of platelets and released during platelet aggregation in haemostasis; chemotactic for monocyte/macrophages and neutrophils; mitogenic for mesodermal cells such as smooth muscle cells, microglia and fibroblasts; similar or identical factors produced by macrophages, endothelial cells, smooth muscle cells and transformed fibroblasts |
| TGF-β (transforming growth factor-β) | Produced by transformed cells in culture; found in platelet α-granules and the gene is induced in activated lymphocytes; induces granulation tissue |
| TNF (tumour necrosis factor or cachexin) | Produced mainly by monocyte/macrophages but also by T-lymphocytes; induced by endotoxin and Gram-positive cell wall products; mediator of general inflammation causing fever and production of IL-1, IL-6 and IL-8 |
| Interleukins | IL-1 initiates granuloma formation in synergy with TNF; IL-2 increases size of granulomas; IL-6 induces acute phase proteins in hepatocytes and stimulates the final differentiation of B-cells; IL-8 induces neutrophil chemotaxis, shape change and granule exocytosis as well as vascular leakage and increased expression of CD-11/CD-18; IL-1 receptor antagonist blocks the effects of IL-1, produced by monocyte/macrophages by the same stimuli that induce IL-1 and presumably limits the effects of IL-1 |

Pusztal L., Lewis C.E., Lorenzen J. and McGee J.O'D (1993) Growth factors: regulation of normal and neoplastic growth. *J. Pathol.*, **169**, 191–201.

van Deuren M., Dofferhoff A.S.M. and van der Meer J.W.M. (1992) Cytokines and the response to infection. *J. Pathol.*, **168**, 349–356.

Hughes S.E. and Hall P.A. (1993) The fibroblast growth factor and receptor multigene families. *J. Pathol.*, **170**, 219–221.

Sawhney N. and Hall P.A. (1992) Ki67 – Structure, function and new antibodies. *J. Pathol.*, **168**, 161–162.

(c) PDGF causes proliferation of dermal myofibroblasts which are then stimulated to produce collagen and fibronectin by TGF-β;

(d) the abnormal expression or overexpression of these growth factors and their cell and nuclear membrane receptors is seen in both infectious and neoplastic situations (*Table 3.1*).

## Definitions

Autocrine = a growth factor that acts upon the cell that produces it.

Paracrine = a growth factor that acts upon another cell, usually close by.

Endocrine = a hormone secreted into the blood and acting on cells which might be at a great distance.

Hyperplasia = increase in size due to increase in cell numbers (reversible when stimulus removed).

Hypertrophy = increase in size due to increase in size of cells (reversible when stimulus removed).

Atrophy = decrease in size due to loss of cells/size of cells (reversible, in principle, when stimulus removed but not true for heart and brain neurones).

Metaplasia = change from one adult cell type to another adult cell type (reversible when stimulus removed).

Neoplasia = mutation to a benign or malignant neoplasm (not reversible).

Dysplasia = altered appearance of cells, which resembles malignant neoplasia but for some reason falls short of true malignancy because it cannot invade or has not yet invaded.

Anaplasia = severe degree of malignant appearance such that the cell of origin is no longer apparent.

## Hyperplasia

- Physiological: breast growth in females at puberty; breast and uterine growth in pregnancy; compensatory hyperplasia in removal of part (liver) or one of a pair of organs (kidney).
- Associated with sequential increased expression of *c-fos*, *c-myc*, *c-ras*.
- Pathological: endometrial hyperplasia; hyperplasia associated with wart virus; prostatic hyperplasia.

# Hypertrophy

- Physiological: striated muscle bulk in training; uterine growth in pregnancy.
- Pathological: myocardial hypertrophy in hypertension.

# Atrophy

- Physiological: involution of uterus following pregnancy.
- Pathological: disuse; denervation; diminution of blood supply, etc. There may be reduction in cellular volume but atrophy can also involve *apoptosis*.

# Metaplasia

- In adult tissues there is no physiological equivalent of metaplasia.
- Examples of metaplasia include: replacement of ciliated columnar cells in the bronchus by squamous cells due to smoke or pollution inhalation; transformation of transitional epithelium to squamous epithelium in the bladder when exposed to stones or *Schistosome* eggs.

# Morphogenesis

- Morphogenesis is the embryonic mass movement of cells as they rearrange to bring tissues into contact for the subsequent process of organogenesis.
- Disruptions at this stage will generally result in non-viable embryos.

# Differentiation

- Differentiation is the process by which an unspecialized cell becomes specialized morphologically, functionally or both.
- In the developing fetus this process underlies the development of distinct cell types, tissues and organs from one totipotent fertilized ovum.
- In the adult some specialized cells are constantly being lost and replaced from a pool of multipotent or unipotent stem cells (haematogenous cells in the bone marrow, skin and gut epithelia).

- The process of differentiation of cells occurs by differential expression and suppression of gene activity not by loss of genes (loss of genes occurs in some other species).
- Organ development occurs in the fourth to eighth weeks and teratogens have the greatest malformation effects at this time (*Table 3.2*).
- Differentiation has a different but related meaning in neoplasia where it refers to the degree of similarity of the cancer cell to the normal equivalent cells.
- In repair processes, such as wound healing, highly differentiated cells such as hair follicles and sweat glands can contribute to the regeneration of the epidermis.
- Less differentiated tissues, such as renal tubules, can regenerate but complex structures, such as glomeruli, cannot.

Braunstein G.D. (1993) Gynecomastia. *N. Engl. J. Med.*, **328**, 490–495.

**Table 3.2  Some human teratogens**

| Agents | Most common abnormalities |
| --- | --- |
| Alcohol | Fetal alcohol syndrome; intrauterine growth retardation (IUGR); microcephaly, ocular and joint anomalies |
| Lithium carbonate | Heart and great vessel anomalies |
| Thalidomide | Limb anomalies (meromelia and amelia); cardiac and kidney defects |
| HIV (human-immunodeficiency virus) | Growth failure; microcephaly; prominent forehead, flattened nasal bridge |
| Rubella | IUGR; cardiac and great vessel anomalies; sensorineural deafness, cataract |

# Cysts

- Cysts are hollow, closed, epithelial-lined structures.
- They are formed in a variety of ways and contain a variety of different materials.

## Skin cysts

- *Implantation cysts* are formed when epidermis is trapped in the dermis either due to trauma or to entrapment during development.

- *Implantation cysts due to entrapment* occur at lines of embryological closure. They are distinguished from other epidermal cysts by having adnexae in their walls.
- *Epidermal and pilar cysts* (commonly and incorrectly called sebaceous cysts) are benign neoplasms of the epithelium of the hair follicle.
- *Inclusion, epidermal and pilar cysts* contain keratin (not sebum) and they may rupture causing a florid, chronic, inflammatory reaction with many giant cells typical of the reaction to keratin in the dermis.
- *Other adnexal tumours* often contain cystic areas as the tumour recapitulates the development of the hollow adnexae.

## Renal cysts

- There are many different types of renal cysts, arising by different mechanisms.
- *Congenital*: the two main syndromes of renal polycystic disease include the *juvenile* (recessive) form and the *adult* (dominant) form.
- It has been said that these arise due to failure of fusion of glomeruli and tubules but the cysts are also found in the liver and pancreas.
- Various *benign cysts* occur with increasing age but also with renal failure; they appear to be the result of post-inflammatory blockage.

## Breast

- Benign breast change (previously called fibrocystic disease, fibro-adenosis and many other terms) may have a mainly cystic presentation.
- Cysts may also arise from other causes such as lactation, galactocele, cystadenoma and retention cysts of the glands of Montgomery.

## Hydatid cysts of the liver (and lung, brain, bone and kidney)

- The life cycle of *Echinococcus granulosus* passes from dogs to sheep, and man is only incidentally involved by eating sheep flesh.
- The cyst consists of a fibrous adventitia which is the host reaction, white elastic laminations derived from the cyst itself and a germinal epithelium on which the brood capsules develop.

## Other cysts

- Many cysts may become secondarily infected and lose their epithelium when they can no longer strictly be called cysts but have become abscesses.
- The ovaries produce a number of physiological cysts, which can sometimes prove a surgical problem.
- The ovary is also covered by a layer of peritoneum and can produce a variety of benign and malignant cysts, many of which may be multilocular.

# 4

# Inflammation, repair and wound healing

## Inflammation

- Inflammation is a stereotyped response to injury.
- In most cases it resolves rapidly but it may persist and become a specifically recognizable chronic entity.
- 'Acute' and 'chronic' refer to the time-course of the process:
    (a) acute inflammation develops rapidly and resolves rapidly;
    (b) chronic inflammation is long-standing.
- Most short-term inflammation has a typical *acute* appearance (mostly neutrophils).
- Most long-standing inflammation has a typical *chronic* appearance (lymphocytes, macrophages, fibroblasts and fibrosis).
- Some inflammatory reactions, however, show *chronic* cells from very early on (tuberculosis) and some long-standing conditions show *acute* cells even after years (chronic osteomyelitis).
- The five classic features of inflammation are:
    (a) redness (rubor);
    (b) heat (calor);
    (c) pain (dolor);
    (d) swelling (tumor);
    (e) loss of function.
- These were first described in the skin by Celsus and, apart from the fifth one which was added later, are mainly a result of vascular dilatation.
- The heat that is evident is only that of the core body temperature since the skin is normally colder than this; an inflamed appendix is only as hot as the other viscera.
- The first step in inflammation is vascular dilatation and all else follows from this.

## Acute inflammation

- The typical features of acute inflammation are well demonstrated in transient trauma to the skin.

- This causes an initial transient (seconds) vasoconstriction followed by vasodilatation of arterioles and capillaries and a variable degree of capillary proliferation (granulation tissue; this does *not* contain granulomas) dependent upon the amount of tissue loss.
- The initial dilatation allows small proteins, such as immunoglobulins, to escape.
- This is followed by further dilatation, which allows larger molecules, such as fibrinogen and plasma proteins, into the wound.
- The dilatation also results in fluid loss into the tissue causing swelling (oedema) and slowing of the blood (stasis) increasing the length of time that various blood-borne factors are in contact with the wound and promoting settling of leukocytes onto vessel walls (margination or pavementing).
- As the dilatation increases, white cells begin to emerge by squeezing between the endothelial junctions (emigration); red cells may also escape in a similar way (diapedesis).

**Table 4.1 Chemical mediators of inflammation**

| Mediators | Source | Release and actions |
| --- | --- | --- |
| *Cellular* Cationic proteins and neutral proteases | Lysosomes in neutrophils | Neutrophils release lysosomal contents in contact with bacteria and damaged tissues, they increase permeability and activate complement |
| Cytokines (including the lymphokines) | These were first described in lymphocytes (hence lymphokines) but are substances produced by many cells that influence other cells | See *Figure 4.1* for their relationships in inflammation |
| Histamine | Mast cells, basophils, eosinophils and platelets | Release is stimulated by C3a, C5a and neutrophil lysosomal proteins, resulting in vasodilatation and transiently increased vascular permeability |
| Leukotrienes | Neutrophils, mast cells, basophils and some macrophages contain the lipoxygenase pathway, which converts arachidonic acid to various leukotrienes; a mixture of these forms slow-reacting substance of anaphylaxis (SRS-A) | The various cells are activated by interleukins and other products of inflammation to secrete leukotrienes some of which ($B_4$) are potent chemoattractants for neutrophils, monocytes and macrophages, while others (SRS-A) cause contraction of smooth muscle and enhance vascular permeability |

**Table 4.1** *continued.*

| Mediators | Source | Release and actions |
|---|---|---|
| Prostaglandins | Cells contain cyclooxygenase which makes prostaglandins from arachidonic acid. Platelets produce thromboxane $A_2$; endothelial cells produce prostacyclin; monocyte/macrophages produce any or all | |
| Nitric oxide | Also known as endothelium-derived relaxing factor, it is a short-lived free radical produced by endothelium and macrophages | It is toxic to bacteria and appears to be a major factor in endotoxic shock |
| *Plasma factors* | | |
| Coagulation proteins | Mostly synthesized in the liver in inactive form; when activated they release fibrin | Intermediates such as FXII are involved in activating other systems but the release of fibrin is an important part of inflammation |
| Complement | Series of 20 proteins synthesized in the liver and in macrophages; the liver produces most but macrophage complement is probably significant at sites of inflammation. The various components form an enzymatic cascade, providing vast ampli-fication of the initial effect | See *Figures 4.2* and *4.3* |
| Fibrinolytic proteins | Mostly synthesized in the liver, they are the negative feedback arm that limits coagulation | Plasmin, which is released by the action of activated FXII, lyses fibrin clot to fibrin degradation products (FDP) |
| Kinins | Circulating clotting factor XII (Hageman factor), prekallikrein and plasminogen are synthesized in the liver and circulate as inactive plasma proteins | FXII is activated by negatively charged surfaces such as exposed basement membranes, proteolytic enzymes, bacterial lipopoly-saccharide (LPS) and foreign materials such as crystals. It converts plasminogen to plasmin and prekallikrein to kallikrein, which, in turn, cleaves kininogen to release bradykinin. It also activates the alternative complement pathway |

Springall D.R. (1995) Nitric oxide – friend and foe. *J. Pathol.*, **175**, 165–166.
Galli S.J. (1993) New concepts about the mast cell. *N. Engl. J. Med.*, **328**, 257–265.

- The white cells move through the tissue to the site of inflammation attracted by the chemical mediators, which are more concentrated the closer they get to the inflammatory site (they ascend a chemical gradient); this process is called chemotaxis.
- Inflammatory cells also show increased random movement in the presence of some mediators (chemokinesis), which increases their statistical chance of encountering sites for their actions.
- Dilatation of vessels also increases the number of red cells in the area, with an increase in oxygen tension for oxygen-dependent free radical killing of infective organisms.
- Damage to local cells results in the release of endogenous chemical mediators as detailed in *Table 4.1* and illustrated in *Figures 4.1–4.3*.
- The lymphatics are also dilated and their physiological role is to return tissue fluid to the venous system, but on the way this is filtered by the lymph nodes and lymphoid cells are exposed to antigens

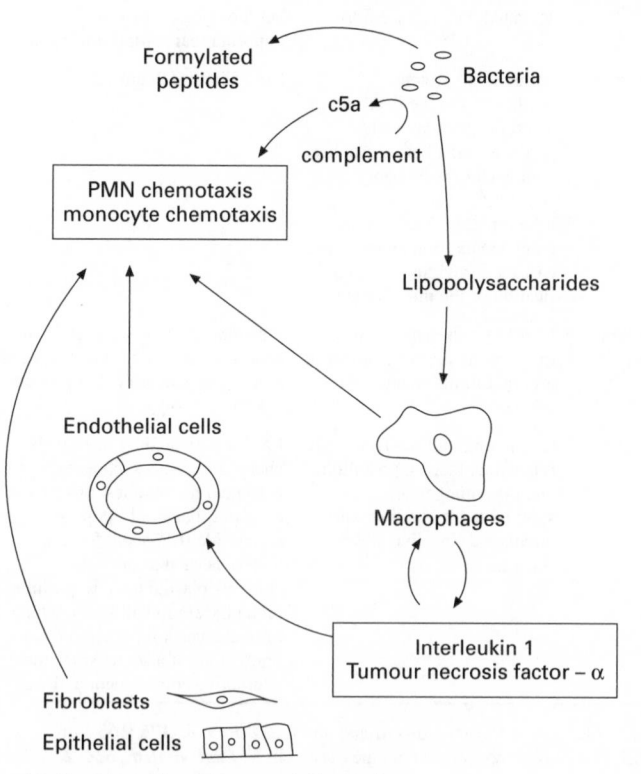

**Figure 4.1** Cytokine pathways in acute inflammation

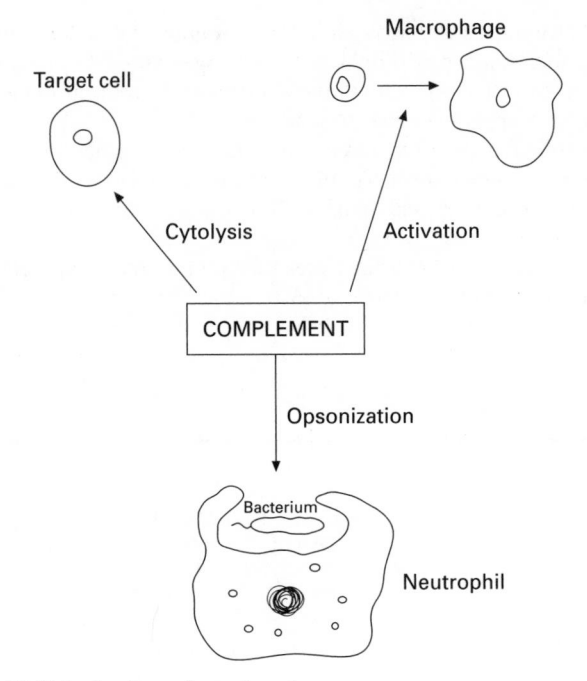

**Figure 4.2** Major functions of complement

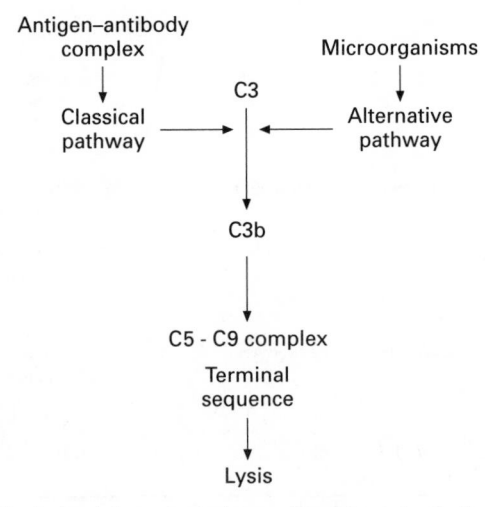

**Figure 4.3** Classical and alternative pathways of complement activation

which stimulates the activation of the immune response. Increased lymphatic drainage also reduces the damage caused by oedema.
- In mild cases the whole process takes about 15 min; in more severe cases it occurs almost instantaneously.
- Following the physical effects that lead to margination, specific cellular binding molecules (called adhesion molecules) are expressed on both circulating and fixed cells causing these to bind together (*Table 4.2*).
- Fluids may collect in various sites that are inflamed and their nature may differ from site to site.

**Table 4.2  Adhesion molecule**

| Adhesion molecule | Cell | Binding site |
|---|---|---|
| *Selectins* | Have extracellular N-terminal domain related to mammalian sugar-binding sites so presumably bind to sugars on other cells | |
| E-selectin (ELAM-1) | Expressed on endothelium | Receptors on leukocytes |
| P-selectin (GMP 140) | Expressed on endothelium and platelets | Receptors on PMNs, monocytes and lymphocytes |
| L-selectin (LAM-1) | Expressed on most leukocyte types and is part of the lymphocyte homing mechanism | High endothelial vessels (HEV) in peripheral lymph nodes |
| *Immunoglobulin family* | | |
| Intercellular adhesion molecule-1 (ICAM-1) | Endothelium | React with integrins found on leukocytes |
| Vascular cell adhesion molecule-1 (VCAM-1) | Endothelium | React with integrins found on leukocytes |
| *Integrins* | | |
| Leukocyte-function-associated antigen-1 (LFA-1) | Leukocytes | Binds to ICAM-1 on endothelium |
| Very late antigen-4 (VLA-4) | Memory T-cells | Binds to VCAM-1 |
| Complement receptor-3 (CR3 or MAC-1) | Monocytes | Binds to ICAM-1 |

PMN, polymorphonucleocyte.

## Definitions

Effusion = fluid collection in a body cavity.

Transudate = low protein oedema fluid (s.g. < 0.015).

Exudate = high protein oedema fluid (s.g. > 0.015) often contains cells and occurs early in mild inflammation.

Serous exudate = no cells and is straw-coloured.

Serosanguinous exudate = serous exudate with red blood cells in it.

Fibrinous exudate = serous exudate with large amounts of fibrin; often deposits on pleural, peritoneal and pericardial surfaces.

Purulent exudate/effusion = contains polymorphs, usually associated with pyogenic bacterial infections.

Suppurative inflammation = purulent exudate associated with liquefactive necrosis.

## Special cases of acute inflammation

### Infections

- Bacteria release exotoxin (or endotoxin as they are damaged) and this causes further vascular dilatation.
- Endotoxin induces interleukin-1 (IL-1) production from the liver and this causes fever (fever may be adaptive since many bacteria have a very narrow range of temperatures at which they can survive).
- If the infection is one that the patient has encountered before, then specific antibodies attach to the organism causing activation of the complement cascade and attack by neutrophils and macrophages, which releases more bacterial fragments and antigens, amplifying the response.
- If the concentration of circulating neutrophils is reduced by this emigration the bone marrow senses this and responds by the production and release of more neutrophils.
- Opsonization involves specific molecules, which bind to bacterial surfaces and render them more likely to be engulfed by phagocytic cells. The main ones are (IgG) and C3b, which are recognized by receptors on the surface of the phagocytic cells, which then ingest them.
- Because there is vasodilatation if the bacteria are not efficiently killed at the periphery, then they may enter the bloodstream as a bacteraemia. If they begin to multiply in the bloodstream, this is a septicaemia.
- If the infection is not resolved locally, then chronic inflammation may wall it off as an abscess. It is said that coagulase positive *Staphylococus aureus* predisposes to abscess formation due to the action of coagulase in causing fibrinogen to produce a fibrin clot.

- If the body encounters this organism again the response is stronger, more rapid and more effective.

van Deuren M., Dofferhoff A.S.M. and van der Meer J.W.M. (1992) Cytokines and the response to infection. *J. Pathol.*, **168**, 349–356.

## Burns

- The depth of burns determines whether an inflammatory response occurs.
- *Superficial burns,* only involving the epidermis, will produce a marked inflammatory reaction.
- *Deeper burns,* which destroy dermal vessels, will not show any clinical inflammation and will have no ability to regenerate and will require grafting to minimize scarring and contractures.
- Beneath the skin damaged muscle will be initiating its own inflammatory response.

## Bedsores (decubitus ulcers)

- Bedsores are pressure ulcers formed in immobile patients.
- They can be very deep and become secondarily infected.
- They predispose to septicaemia and death.
- Prevention is a matter of good nursing care, involving regular moving and turning the patient and careful skin care including massage to increase blood flow to the area; but with poor peripheral perfusion in terminally ill patients bedsores may be unavoidable as a pre-terminal event.
- Skin over bony prominences can be protected by foam rubber or sheepskins and 'ripple beds' may be used.

## Hypersensitivity reactions

- Altered responsiveness can result in excessive or inappropriate reactions, which can trigger an acute inflammatory reaction.

## Treatment

- The role of inflammation is to deal with damage and to facilitate regeneration or to begin repair if regeneration is not possible or is restricted.
- Treatment is directed at the causes (antibiotics in bacterial infections).
- Many of the features of inflammation are unpleasant for the patient and pain should always be adequately treated, but inflammation is

beneficial in most cases and simple suppression of it is counter-productive.

## Chronic inflammation

- Chronic inflammation arises in unresolved acute inflammation or very early (*ab initio*) in the inflammatory response in some special circumstances such as tuberculosis or sterile foreign bodies.
- It contains characteristic cells (lymphocytes, epithelioid cells, macrophages, giant cells, fibroblasts) and structures such as granulomas and fibrosis.
- The varying proportions of these components allow further subclassification of chronic inflammation into several types, some of which are characteristic of specific diseases.
- Chronic inflammation is also characterized by more extensive tissue destruction than is typical in acute inflammation due to the lengthy nature of the process and the greater lysosomal rupture with the release of numerous lytic enzymes.
- Hypersensitivity plays a significant role in chronic inflammation and the greater the inflammatory response then the greater the tissue damage in many situations, for example:
  - (a) lepromatous leprosy: little immune response, many bacteria in the skin and nasal secretions, little tissue damage, patients eventually die;
  - (b) tuberculoid leprosy: strong immune response, few bacteria found, great tissue destruction but patients survive.
- The change from the typical, acute, cellular infiltrate to a chronic pattern is due to the actions of a series of cytokines, complement fractions and factors from the initiating agent, often modified by the inflammatory cells.
- Macrophages accumulate in the area due to migration inhibition factor.

### Definitions

Macrophages = cells from the macrophage monocyte series; in tissues they are also called histiocytes, and in the circulation, monocytes.

Epithelioid cells = transformed macrophages whose metabolism is dominated by secretion and no longer by ingestion; they look epithelial.

Giant cells = cells with one cytoplasm but several nuclei (*Table 4.3*).

Fibroblasts = spindle-shaped cells of the connective tissue which produce various polysaccharides, collagens and elastin (they do *not* produce fibrin, which comes from the liver as fibrinogen).

**Table 4.3. Types of giant cells**

| Giant cells | Features | Occurrence |
|---|---|---|
| *Pathological* | | |
| Foreign body | Nuclei arranged randomly | Inflammatory reactions where the foreign body cannot be ingested by single macrophages |
| Langhans* | Nuclei arranged as a horseshoe at one end | Tuberculosis and other mycobacterial infections |
| Touton | Nuclei arranged in a circle towards the centre with fat containing foamy cytoplasm around them | Inflammatory reactions containing fat, also in histiocytic tumours |
| Tumour | Bizarre nuclei | Usually in anaplastic carcinomas |
| Viral | Giant nuclei with nuclear and cytoplasmic inclusions | Warthin–Finkeldey cells in measles |
| Reed–Sternberg | Double nucleus | Hodgkin's lymphoma |
| *Physiological* | | |
| Megakaryocytes | Random nuclei | In bone marrow, platelets are fragments of the cytoplasm alone |
| Osteoclasts | Random nuclei | Along bony surfaces in the marrow where bone resorption is occurring |
| *Syncytial* | | |
| Cardiac muscle | Branching and fusing cytoplasm | Normal myocardium |
| Syncytiotrophoblast | Giant syncytium often surrounding villi | Normal pregnancy |

* Langhans' giant cell should not be confused with Langerhans' dendritic cells of the epidermis.

## Types of chronic inflammatory reactions

- *Chronic inflammation as a primary response*: some diseases cause little or no acute inflammatory phase because their initiation is due to cell-mediated immunological mechanisms.
- *Autoimmune diseases* are generally lymphocytic from the beginning although the initiating step may sometimes be bacterial and the reaction to that phase is acute in type.
- *Viral infections* are often chronic *ab initio*.
- *Parasitic infections* may stimulate a primarily chronic response,

although they are also characterized by local and circulatory eosinophilia.
- *Tumours* frequently evoke inflammation and this is mainly chronic in nature.
- *Acute inflammation leading to chronic inflammation*:
  (a) this is chronic inflammation in which the preceding acute, inflammatory response cannot deal with some or all of the initial insult;
  (b) foreign body reactions are like this and may also rapidly develop into granulomatous reactions.
- *Granulomatous inflammation*:
  (a) some forms of chronic inflammation are characterized by more or less ordered assemblages of transformed macrophages called granulomas (*Table 4.4*);
  (b) the granulomas consist of separate macrophages but may be accompanied by giant cells;
  (c) transformed macrophages look like epithelial cells and are often called epithelioid macrophages;
  (d) they have extensive cytoplasm containing rough endoplasmic reticulum (ER), Golgi apparatus and numerous vesicles which are not lysosomes;
  (e) epithelioid macrophages are protein-producing cells and have a reduced ability to phagocytose but can produce a wide variety of chemical mediators;

**Table 4.4  Types of granulomas**

| Type of granuloma | Appearances |
| --- | --- |
| Sarcoid | Small collection of epithelioid macrophages, no lymphocytes (naked granuloma) |
| Tuberculous | The most highly structured of granulomas; central, caseous necrosis, surrounded by epithelioid macrophages with Langhans' giant cells and an outer surround of lymphocytes |
| Foreign body | Loose type of granuloma with many foreign body giant cells, often containing debris |
| Crohn's | Chronic inflammatory bowel disease with fistulae, can also occur in skin, must be distinguished from the foreign body granulomas that can occur in bowel damage generally |
| Palisading granulomas | Collections of macrophages and lymphocytes surrounding altered collagen, commonly in the skin in rheumatoid disease, granuloma annulare and necrobiosis lipoidica (often in association with diabetes mellitus) |

Sheffield E.A. (1990) The granulomatous inflammatory response. *J. Pathol.*, **160**, 1–2.

(f) macrophages can divide in peripheral sites but most are recruited from the circulation as monocytes which then become tissue macrophages; they can fuse in the periphery forming giant cells;

(g) cytoskeletal structures can sometimes be seen at light microscopy (asteroid bodies);

(h) lysosomal debris can sometimes be seen (Schaumann bodies);

(i) many granulomas form under the influence of delayed hyper-sensitivity to the inciting antigen but granulomas in sarcoidosis do not seem to involve this;

(j) IL-1 is capable of inducing granuloma formation in humans;

(k) granulomas are found in a variety of conditions:
- (i) beryllium and zirconium sensitivity
- (ii) foreign body reactions
- (iii) sarcoidosis
- (iv) Crohn's disease
- (v) primary biliary cirrhosis
- (vi) tuberculosis
- (vii) leprosy
- (viii) syphilis
- (ix) drugs

## Wound healing

- Inflammation is the first step in wound healing.
- It attempts to deal with the cause, remove debris and provide a frame-work for complete tissue regeneration or repair.
- *Healing by primary intention* refers to incised wounds where the edges can be apposed.
- *Healing by secondary intention* is where there has been tissue loss and the edges cannot be suitably apposed.
- Wound healing by primary intention is rapid (after about 10 days the wound is strong and only remodelling occurs from then on).
- Wound healing by secondary intention is slower since granulation tissue has to form from the base of the wound and re-epithelialization has to occur from the edges to cover this, and eventually the tissue deficit is made good by scar tissue.
- The time-scale depends upon the degree of tissue loss or the extent of the process that prevents apposition.

### Regeneration

- Regeneration refers to the total healing of the wound with restitution of the original tissues in their usual amounts and forms and with normal function.

- To some extent repair depends upon the nature of the tissue that has been damaged, the amount of tissue that has been lost, removal of the injurious agent, the integrity of the healing process and any interruption to the healing process.
- The regenerative capacity of cells varies. Some cells are able to regenerate with ease (labile cells), some to only a limited extent (stable cells) and some cannot regenerate at all (permanent cells).
- Loss of permanent cells can only be repaired by other cells and fibrosis. Loss of stable cells can be replaced to a limited extent. Loss of labile cells can (in principle) be totally regenerated.

## Repair (fibrosis)

- In the presence of severe damage, damage to stable or permanent cells, large tissue deficiencies, or interrupted healing for any reason, a variable degree of repair takes place.
- Repair means that the original tissue is not totally regenerated and the deficit is made good to some extent by fibrosis forming a scar.

Border W.A. and Noble N.A. (1994) Transforming growth factor beta in tissue fibrosis. *N. Engl. J. Med.*, **331**, 1286–1292.

## Delayed healing

- Many materials and processes are required for wound healing to occur properly and deficiencies in any of these can delay or prevent adequate wound healing.
- Although these effects are traditionally divided into local and systemic effects, many (such as blood supply) may be due to either or both.

## Local effects

### Vascular supply

- An intact blood supply is essential for wound healing to occur since the repair of damaged cells in the area is energy-dependent.
- Different areas of the body are better supplied than others (facial wounds heal rapidly, pretibial ones are slow).
- Removal of debris and toxic material also needs intact blood flow.
- The blood carries various inflammatory mediators to the site.
- Lymphatic drainage is essential to remove oedema and to carry antigens to the lymph nodes.
- Healing is relatively poor in territories supplied by vessels affected by atheroma, such as leg ulcers in arteriopaths.

- The significance of blood supply is seen in fractures of the scaphoid where the supply is interrupted and avascular necrosis supervenes.

## Nutrients and oxygen

- The local blood supply determines the delivery of oxygen and nutrients to the site but the general nutritional and respiratory function determines what is available to be brought to the site, thus the elderly and malnourished patients show relatively poor wound healing.

## Infection

- Infection provides a continuing stimulus to inflammation and tissue death and destruction, healing does not occur, for example in chronic osteomyelitis.
- Systemic infection also delays wound healing for reasons that are not clear.
- Infection is much more likely in some surgical sites than in others and a distinction is often drawn between:
    (a) 'clean' operation wounds: subcutaneous lipoma, inguinal hernia;
    (b) 'contaminated' operation wounds: those, other than skin, with a known normal flora such as colon, mouth, vagina;
    (c) 'infected' operation wounds: sites infected at the time of surgery; abscess.

## Foreign material

- Prostheses are always at risk from infection but may also cause delayed wound healing directly (as with comminuted fractures).
- Suture materials and, rarely, swabs left in the patient often interfere with healing.

## Ionizing radiation

- This damages epithelial cells and fibroblast, making wound healing less efficient.
- In the longer term vascular damage makes the tissue less viable.

## Excessive mobility

- Instability of the wound delays healing; this is most noticeable in fractures but skin dehiscence will occur, particularly in the early stages before good scar tissue has formed.

## Systemic factors

### Nutrition

- Protein is needed in the diet because so much of wound healing is dependent upon protein synthesis *de novo,* including cellular enzymes, inflammatory cells, collagen and elastin.
- Vitamin C and copper are essential for collagen synthesis, as is zinc, and this may be lost in burns and intestinal fistulae making treatment of these even more difficult.

### Diabetes mellitus

- Diabetics are more prone to infection but diabetes also impairs wound healing in general.

### Corticosteroid treatment

- Corticosteroids inhibit inflammation and specifically reduce macrophage numbers with consequent lowering of macrophage-derived growth factors.

### Malignancy

- Patients with malignant disease heal badly, probably due to relative cachexia.

## Examples of healing in various tissues

### Skin

- Experimental studies on wound healing have largely been performed on skin and most of our knowledge is derived from this tissue.
- In a sterile incisional wound healing by primary intention there is relatively little cell death and no foreign bodies.
- Within minutes the narrow cut is filled with blood from cut vessels and this clots within seconds to minutes.
- By 24 h neutrophil polymorphs have entered the wound and moved towards the fibrin clot.
- Epidermal cells begin to proliferate at the edges of the cut, causing it to thicken.
- Damaged adnexae (hair follicles and sweat glands) have stem cells within them and these may de-differentiate further to general skin stem cells and contribute to restoring any epidermal deficiency.
- The epithelial cells migrate over the clot surface depositing basement membrane as they go; they fuse beneath the scab.

- By 72 h the neutrophils are replaced by macrophages, granulation tissue replaces the fibrin clot and collagen is forming at the edges.
- Wound contraction occurs due to the myofibroblasts in the granulation tissue reducing the size of the defect by up to 80%.
- The epidermal cells continue to proliferate and become multilayered.
- By day 5 granulation tissue is at its maximum; collagen changes from vertical to horizontal orientation and begins to bridge the wound 'organizing' the granulation tissue; the epidermis has now returned to full thickness (about six cells depending on body site) and is keratinizing.
- After 2 weeks the collagen is remodelling, the new vessels are regressing and the inflammatory infiltrate has largely disappeared.
- After a month the scar is well formed but continues to remodel for some further months and tensile strength continues to increase.
- Tensile strength of collagen is largely a matter of cross-linkages and these form between collagen bundles.
- The degree of scarring depends to some extent on whether the initial wound was parallel or transverse to the major orientation of the collagen bundles (Langer's lines); cutting across the bundles produces far more nodular scars than cutting along them; even better scars are produce by splitting the bundles apart rather than cutting.
- In healing by secondary intention the process of fibrosis and scarring is a more prominent element.
- Some abnormalities of the healing process may occur:
  (a) sometimes the granulation tissue response is so florid that the epithelium does not manage to grow over it and a friable nodule of exuberant granulation tissue protrudes above the surface, often secondarily infected and called a pyogenic granuloma (the older surgeon's 'proud flesh');
  (b) abnormalities in collagen synthesis also occur leading to hypertrophic scars and, in extreme cases, to very florid overgrowths called keloids (most common in people of Afro-Caribbean descent).

## Bone

- Following fracture to a long bone, blood leaks from the ruptured vessels within the bone and from those in the periosteum and a haematoma forms.
- This forms a basis for the migration of cells.
- Polymorphs, macrophages and fibroblasts migrate in over the fibrin meshwork, new vessels form, fibrosis occurs and by the end of the first week the clot is organized.
- Degranulated platelets and migrating inflammatory cells release

platelet-derived growth factor (PDGF), transforming growth factor-$\alpha$ (TGF-$\alpha$) and fibroblast growth factor (FGF).

- Activated periosteal osteoblasts begin to form trabeculae of woven bone and the activated mesenchymal cells in the soft tissues around the fracture transform into chondroblasts and begin to produce fibrocartilage and hyaline cartilage, which envelops the fracture site.
- By weeks 2–3 the repair tissue reaches its maximum girth, although it is still too weak to support weight.
- As the woven bone approaches the new cartilage, this undergoes enchondrial ossification and in this fashion the deficit is bridged by bony callus.
- As the callus matures and begins to transmit weight-bearing stresses, the bone remodels and resorbs non-weight-bearing trabeculae until it may be almost impossible to detect where the fracture had been.

Freemont A.J. (1996) The pathology of osteogenesis imperfecta. *J. Clin. Pathol.*, **49**, 618–619.

## Liver

- The general principles of inflammation and wound healing also apply to the liver but when the injurious agent is not removed, as in persistent viral damage, or autoimmune disease, such as primary biliary cirrhosis or chronic alcohol abuse, then fibrosis comes to dominate the picture and cirrhosis develops.
- Cirrhosis consists of regenerating nodules of hepatocytes surrounded by fibrosis and this disturbs the vascular organization, leading to portal hypertension and thus oesophageal varices.
- Liver function is also disturbed and obstructive jaundice with eventual liver failure is often the cause of death.

## Kidney

- Damage to the kidney follows the same sort of sequence as most inflammatory and healing processes but tubules will regenerate, like many epithelia, if their reticulin pattern remains undamaged, but the more complex glomeruli will not.

## Nervous tissue

- Injury to the brain, resulting in death of neural tissue, cannot be regenerated because the neurones are permanent cells (postmitotic) which can no longer divide.

- Heart muscle is the same and it is possible that it is the complex spatial electrical connections in these two tissues that makes attempts at regeneration too complex.

Slavin J. (1996) The role of cytokines in wound healing. *J. Pathol.*, **178**, 5–10.

# 5

# Immunology and immunopathology

## Immunology

- The immune system works by recognizing foreign molecules.
- When it encounters these it can produce a humoral (antibody) response or a cellular response or both.
- The immune system interacts with a number of other systems including kinins, complement, clotting, thrombolytic and neural.
- Interstitial fluid is returned to the venous circulation by the lymphatics.
- Infections shed proteins into the interstitial fluid, as do tumours.
- In the lymphatic system there are nodules of lymphoid tissue (lymph nodes), which filter the lymph.
- If they encounter foreign molecules (proteins or polysaccharides mainly), they respond to these with an antigenic response.
- Lymph nodes may be resting if unstimulated, reactive, infected, involved by primary tumours or by secondary tumours.
- There are several features of the immune system which are essential for its function; it has to show:
  - (a) specificity: many parasite or infection antigens are very similar and specificity of response is essential;
  - (b) diversity: the immune system has encountered numerous antigens over its evolution but during the lifetime of any one individual it is likely to encounter antigens for which it has no programme and it must have the ability to respond to a great range of antigens that are new to it;
  - (c) memory: the first time that an individual encounters an antigen its response may be slow and relatively non-specific; part of the response will include developing a more rapid and specific response for the next encounter and remembering that;
  - (d) recruitment of other defence systems: the immune system on its own cannot rid the body of all foreign antigens and it therefore produces chemical messengers, which recruit other cellular

systems, such as polymorphs, macrophages and mast cells, as well as complement, kinins and lytic enzymes.

Williams G.T. (1994) Apoptosis in the immune system. *J. Pathol.*, **173**, 1–4.

## Humoral immunity

- Humoral immunity is the production of antibodies, which are small, soluble globulin proteins (immunoglobulins, Ig).
- Antibodies bind to antigens and have different effects depending on where the antigen is and which accessory processes are activated.
- They can:
  (a) cause bacterial lysis;
  (b) neutralize toxins;
  (c) make foreign material more digestible by macrophages (opsonization) and cause antibody-dependent cell-mediated cytotoxicity.
- The production of antibodies is dependent upon differentiation of B-lymphocytes to plasma cells.
- The B-cell receptor is on the surface of the B-cell and the antigen-binding component of this is IgM and the specificity is provided by rearrangements of the immunoglobulin genes.
- All antibodies have a similar structure, with two hypervariable antigen-binding sites (Fab) and a constant region (Fc).
- A plasma cell produces only one specific antibody but in large numbers.
- There are five classes of antibody:
  (a) IgM: this is the first antibody to appear during response to a new antigenic stimulus:
    (i)   J chains connect five IgM molecules together so that it has 10 reactive sites, which makes it efficient at agglutination and complement fixing.
  (b) IgG: this is the antibody found in highest concentration in the plasma:
    (i)   it is characteristic of the secondary immune response;
    (ii)  it can cross the placenta to provide passive immunity to the fetus;
    (iii) it can neutralize toxins and can be indirectly cytotoxic by binding to cells and then activating complement;
    (iv)  polymorphs and macrophages have receptors to the Fc region and IgG can therefore facilitate opsonization.
  (c) IgA: exists as a dimer connected by a J chain:
    (i)   it is secreted by plasma cells at the base of mucosal surfaces which have receptors for dimeric Fc regions and transported

onto the surface by a secretory piece that is then cleaved;
   (ii) it is the major immune protection for mucosal surfaces.
(d) IgE: binds to the surface of mast cells by its Fc portion in anaphylactic type hypersensitized individuals:
   (i) subsequent exposure to the antigen causes binding to the Fab portion which causes the mast cells to degranulate, releasing various inflammatory mediators.
(e) IgD: little is known about this antibody but it is expressed on the surface of some lymphocytes and probably acts in leukocyte recognition.

## Cell-mediated immunity

- The cells are T-lymphocytes.
- T-lymphocytes are characterized by an antigen-specific T-cell receptor (TCR), which is made up of one of two pairs of polypeptide chains ($\alpha$, $\beta$, $\gamma$, $\delta$) and TCR diversity is achieved by somatic variations in these chains.
- There are two main sets of T-lymphocytes:
  (a) helper T-lymphocytes (CD4);
  (b) suppresser/cytotoxic T-lymphocytes (CD8).
- Helper cells respond to antigenic stimulation by producing cytokines which activate other T-cells, B-cells and macrophages.
- Suppresser cells suppress the activity of B-cells and help to regulate B-cell response and also to prevent autoimmune disease.

### Other cells involved in the lymphocyte response

- *Macrophages*: these cells have a significant role in inflammation generally but are also specifically involved with lymphocyte activity:
  (a) They process and present antigen to immunocompetent T-cells since T-cells cannot be activated by soluble antigen;
  (b) they produce a number of cytokines;
  (c) they can lyse tumour cells and may be used by lymphocytes during immune surveillance;
  (d) they will also phagocytose microorganisms, especially when coated with IgG, IgM or C3b.
- *Dendritic and Langerhans' cells*: these are non-phagocytic but possess a large surface area for the presentation of antigens.
- *Natural killer (NK) cells*: lymphocytes with no TCR or cell surface immunoglobulins, they can lyse virus-infected cells, tumour cells and some normal cells without prior sensitization:
  (a) they are said to be part of the 'natural' as opposed to adaptive immune system;

(b) one of the surface markers (CD16) is an Fc receptor for IgG and allows NK cells to lyse IgG-coated target cells (antibody-dependent cytotoxicity).

## Lymphoid system

- Lymph nodes are small reniform nodules scattered through the lymphatic system or arranged in groups at major sites of drainage (axillae, groins, neck, etc.).
- The anatomic distribution of vessels and nodes is less constant than for other structures and very few are named.
- As well as the nodes, there are numerous collections of lymphoid tissue that are not encapsulated (Peyer's patches, etc.), known as the diffuse lymphoid system.
- Collections of lymphoid tissue can also be induced by various means such as long-standing inflammation, thus the stomach has no resident lymphoid tissue but can develop it following long periods of gastritis.
- The tissue-specific lymphocytes circulate but home to that tissue. Tissue specificity of this sort depends upon CD44 markers on the lymphocyte surface.
- The function of lymph nodes is to filter the lymph and to bring it into contact with the blood, since lymph travels from tissue areas to the nodes. The effector cells and antibodies must be delivered to the pathological sites by arteries.
- The function of the spleen is to filter the blood and destroy defunct blood cells and to bring the contents of the blood into contact with lymphoid tissue.
- The function of the thymus is to provide a site for the maturation of T-lymphocytes (thymus-dependent lymphocytes).
- The cells of the lymphoid system are produced in the bone marrow and at a very early stage the T-lymphocytes migrate to the thymus and mature, then leave and populate the lymph nodes and the thymus becomes redundant and atrophies.
- There is no equivalent B-cell maturation anatomical site and these seem to mature in the nodes or the diffuse lymphoid system.

## Lymphadenopathy

- When lymph nodes enlarge and are readily palpable this is called lymphadenopathy regardless of the cause.
- Lymph nodes may enlarge due to:
  (a) reactive changes;
  (b) infection of the lymph node;

    (c) primary malignancy;

    (d) secondary malignancy.

- There are three reactive compartments in the lymph node:

    (a) B-cell areas which are small and uniform in the inactive node (primary follicles) and enlarged (secondary) with centres consisting of large cells (centroblasts and centrocytes) surrounded by small dark- staining cells (B-lymphocytes with a few T-lymphocytes activating or suppressing the B-cell activity);

    (b) the follicle centres also contain various dendritic cells which are presenting antigens to the active lymphocytes and may contain visible material (tingible body macrophages);

    (c) T-cell areas are located between the follicles and consist mainly of T-cells but with a few B-cells, macrophages and dendritic cells;

    (d) beneath the capsule is a sinus which ramifies throughout the node and contains mainly macrophages;

    (e) the fourth structure spreading through the lymph node is high endothelial cell vascular tree which allows traffic of lymphocytes in and out of the bloodstream.

- Any or all of the reactive compartments can be expanded, dependent upon the type of stimulus being received.

- The sinuses are expanded if the node is draining an area in which there is considerable necrosis; the follicles are activated by soluble antigen and the T-zones by viruses and cell-bound antigens.

- The pattern of reaction is sometimes characteristic but is more often only suggestive of specific diseases.

- The afferent lymphatics enter the general surface of the lymph node into the subcapsular sinus and this is therefore the first site at which secondary malignant deposits become established (*Figure 5.1*).

- From the subcapsular area they spread out and eventually replace the whole node and can then breach the capsule and spread into surrounding tissue.

- In the early stages it may be possible to identify cancer cells in the subcapsular sinus of grossly normal nodes but the significance of this is unclear as there is at least some degree of immune surveillance and destruction of cancer cells by immunological means, and it may be that prophylactic removal of nodes removes a barrier to further spread. In the case of established nodal metastasis there is presumably less doubt.

- Primary tumours of lymphoid tissue are termed lymphomas but this term implies benignancy whereas most are malignant and should be called lymphosarcomas.

- There are numerous different lymphomas and almost as many classifications; the most straightforward system is to classify the non-

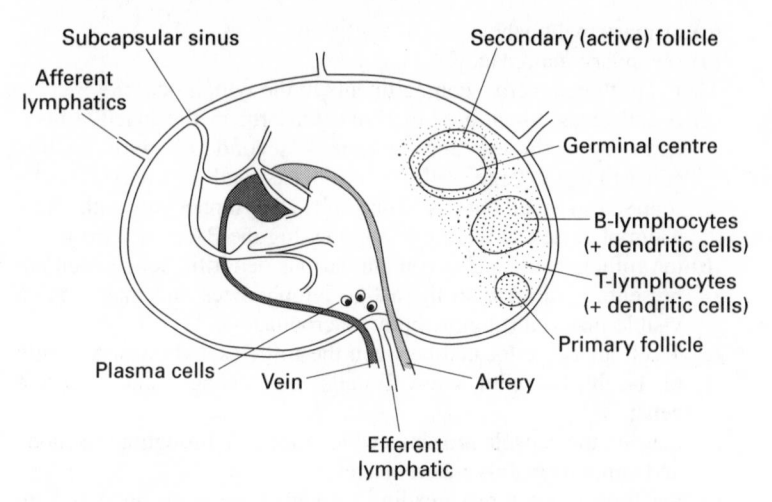

**Figure 5.1** Diagram of a lymph node illustrating the functional contact between blood, lymph and lymphoid tissue

Hodgkin's lymphomas on the basis of their resemblance to the normal constituents of lymph nodes after separating Hodgkin's lymphoma first.

- The extranodal lymphomas are classified separately. Lymphomas are primary to the lymph nodes and also they do not appear first in the subcapsular sinus but in the general body of the node and are often difficult to identify.
- The mainstay of lymphoma diagnosis and classification is immuno-cytochemistry of the highly specific cell surface molecules and the molecular genetics of these. These are so specific that lymphomas have been the most convincingly classified and extensively investigated human malignancies.
- In the process of draining infected areas the lymph nodes themselves may become infected (often showing polymorphs) and some infections, often viral, specifically involve lymphoid tissue.
- Infections such as cat scratch fever, infectious mononucleosis and human immunodeficiency virus (HIV) specifically attack lymphoid tissue, giving lymphadenopathy as one of the signs.
- The lymphatic vessels leading to the lymph nodes may also become involved in disease, particularly infection, and the red lines of lymphangitis leading to enlarged infected or reactive nodes are a clear clinical indication of this.

Isaacson P.G. and Spencer J. (1995) The biology of low grade MALT lymphoma. *J. Clin. Pathol.*, **48**, 395–397.

## Hypersensitivity reactions

- Hypersensitivity is a state of altered immunological responsiveness in which a severe or harmful reaction occurs on exposure to an allergen.
- The reactions only occur in sensitized individuals and so cannot occur on the first exposure.
- Four (or sometimes five) types of hypersensitivity are described:
  - (a) *type I (anaphylactic or immediate)*: this reaction occurs within minutes of exposure to the antigen and is the basic mechanism in most types of childhood eczema, hayfever and extrinsic asthma:
    - (i) the precipitating agents such as pollens are often introduced in small amounts causing local effects but systemic applications of penicillin or other drugs may cause severe symptoms of anaphylaxis which can result in death;
    - (ii) the process is mediated by IgE.
  - (b) *type II (cytotoxic)*: the binding of IgG or IgM antibodies to cell surfaces resulting in lymphocytic, macrophage or complement lysis of the cell:
    - (i) this can be detected using the Coombs' test, which uses rabbit antihuman immunoglobulin to agglutinate the affected cells;
    - (ii) it is the underlying mechanism of idiopathic thrombo-cytopenic purpura and rhesus incompatibility, causing hydrops fetalis in rhesus mismatch.
  - (c) *type III (immune complex)*: large amounts of antigen–antibody complexes can deposit in various tissues and cause complement activation and tissue destruction, as with the acute diffuse proliferative glomerulonephritis associated with beta haemolytic streptococcal sore throat:
    - (i) some of the damage in rheumatoid arthritis, polyarteritis nodosa and systemic lupus erythematosus (SLE) is also antigen–antibody associated.
  - (d) *type IV (delayed)*: cell-mediated hypersensitivity involving specifically primed T-lymphocytes:
    - (i) the reaction takes typically 12–24 h to develop;
    - (ii) it is concerned with the response to viruses, fungi and some bacteria such as mycobacteria;
    - (iii) it is also involved in delayed skin contact hypersensitivity, autoimmune disease and the reaction to altered epitopes on tumour cells;

(iv) the reaction is initiated by helper T-cells which recognize alien epitopes on the cell surface of antigen-presenting cells in conjunction with host class II HLA molecules. The lymphocytes secrete lymphokines which attract T cytotoxic and suppressor cells to the area and result in cell lysis.

(e) *'Type V' (stimulatory)*: the only well-established version of this type of hypersensitivity is in Graves' disease, in which antibodies to thyroid-stimulating hormone (TSH) receptors on the thyroid cells cause stimulation or blockage of the functions of these receptors (growth or activation of the thyroid cells):

(i)  the long-acting thyroid stimulator is an IgG antibody.

# Immunodeficiency

There are non-specific and specific immunodeficiencies.

* *Non-specific deficiencies* involve systems such as the neutrophil deficiencies, defects in complement and some systemic diseases which make intact, specific immune responses ineffective.
* *Specific deficiencies* are defects in the immune system itself and these are classified as primary (usually genetic) and secondary (acquired).
* Primary deficiencies include:
  (a) X-linked agammaglobulinaemia (of Bruton), which is one of the most common and presents at a few months of age when maternal immunoglobulins have been used up. The children develop mainly pyogenic infections such as staphylococcal and *Haemophilus influenzae* infections; they have no circulating immunoglobulins except for occasional low levels of IgG;
  (b) the genetic defect is a specific B-cell tyrosine kinase molecule.
* Common variable immunodeficiency is a fairly common but heterogeneous condition in which the common features are a relative agammaglobulinaemia due to the inability of B-cells to differentiate into plasma cells.
* Isolated IgA deficiency occurs in about 1:600 Europeans and can be inherited or acquired as a result of some viral infections:
  (a) the significance of the condition is a matter of debate but the abnormality is an inability of IgA lymphocytes to mature.
* Thymic hypoplasia (DiGeorge's syndrome) is a congenital abnormality brought about by the failure of development of the third and fourth pharyngeal pouches with resultant lack of thymus and parathyroids:
  (a) patients lack T-cells and are prone to fungal and viral infections.
* Severe combined immunodeficiency disease (SCID) has both B- and

T-cell deficiencies and affected infants are prone to a wide range of bacterial, viral and fungal infections:
  (a) it is a heterogeneous collection of diseases and some are effectively treated with bone marrow transplant

Rosen F.S., Cooper M.D. and Wedgwood R.J. (1995) The primary immunodeficiencies. *N. Engl. J. Med.*, **333**, 431–440.

* Secondary immunodeficiency is dominated by the effects of HIV:
  (a) the full expression is the acquired immuno deficiency syndrome (AIDS), with numerous infections as a result of suppression of cell- mediated immunity (particularly CD44+ T-cells).

# Transplant immunology

* The basic fact of transplant immunology was recognized in the fact that skin transplants in mice survived longer in animals that were more closely related.
* Transplant immunology is mainly a function of HLA types: the closer these are, the better the chance of graft survival.

## Definitions

Autograft = graft and host the same animal.
Isograft = donor and host from the same inbred strain (monozygous twins excepted).
Allograft = donor and host same species but not genetically identical.
Xenograft = donor and host different species.
Major histocompatibility complex (MHC) = the general term for the closely related set of genes coding for a series of cell surface and plasma protein antigens.
Human leukocyte antigen (HLA) = the human version of MHC located on the short arm of chromosome 6.

## HLA system

* Obviously the HLA system did not evolve to control transplantation, which is not a natural event.
* HLA gene products are a heterogeneous set of recognition molecules for lymphocytes.
* The genes are carried on the short arm of chromosome 6 and code for three classes of molecule:
  (a) class I: these encode the heavy chains of a group of antigens which include the classic transplantation antigens:

(i)  the gene product is an α–glycoprotein transmembrane molecule non-covalently bound to a β-chain (a $\beta_2$-microglobulin) unrelated to the HLA complex and coded on chromosome 15;

(ii)  the class I genes are arranged in B, C, A regions.

(b)  class II: these consist of a pair of non-covalently bound α and β dimers, both of which have transmembrane domains:

(i)  class II genes include four D regions (DP, DQ, DR, DZ) which are further subdivided into 13 subtypes.

Both class I and II are part of the superfamily of molecules that include immunoglobulins, T-cell surface antigens CD4 and CD8 as well as T-cell antigen receptor.

(c)  class III: these genes code for components of the complement system.

- These genes are interspersed with other, apparently unrelated, genes.
- Helper and suppressor T-cells recognize foreign antigen in association with class II histocompatability antigens on antigen-presenting cells.
- Cytotoxic T-cells recognize class I antigens together with viral antigens on most somatic cells.
- As well as determining matches in transplantations the HLA subtypes are statistically related to various diseases.
- The association is variable ranging from 100% in HLA-DR2 in narcolepsy to a 2–3 times relative risk with B8 and B15 in insulin-dependent diabetes mellitus.

Dick H.M. and Powis S.H. (1987) HLA and disease: possible mechanisms. *Recent Adv. Histopathol.*, **13**, 1–12.

## Transplant rejection

- Transplant rejection is often classified on the basis of its time-course:
  - (a)  *hyperacute*: within minutes and due to preformed cytotoxic antibodies to donor antigens particularly blood group substances;
  - (b)  *accelerated*: 2–4 days; previous sensitization to donor antigens often due to previous transplants;
  - (c)  *acute*: 1–3 weeks; cellular response to donor antigens;
  - (d)  chronic; more than 3 months due to breakdown of tolerance.
- Graft-versus-host disease (GVHD) occurs when immunocompetent lymphocytes are introduced into an immunocompromised  host in sufficient numbers; this generally only occurs in bone transplants and results in various disease states: diarrhoea; dermatitis; anaemia; cholestatic liver disease. Death may occur in severe cases.

Sloane J.P. and Norton J. (1993) The pathology of bone marrow transplantation. *Histopathology*, **22**, 201–209.

Appleton A.L. and Sviland L. (1993) Current thoughts on the pathogenesis of graft versus host disease. *J. Clin. Pathol.*, **46**, 785–789.

# Tumour immunology

- In histological preparations of tumours there are often a large number of lymphocytes in the vicinity and the draining lymph nodes often seem to be making a brisk response, with B-cell, T-cell and sinusoidal activation, and there is some evidence that breast cancer prognosis is related to these, but strong proof is still lacking.
- Many cancers seem to be able to colonize lymph nodes and to thrive there. Regression in some tumours is well described and occasionally this can be spontaneous and complete.
- Some workers claim to induce cancer regression by non-specific stimulation of the immune system with Bacille Calmette-Guérin (BCG) and other immunogens.
- Some cancers have been shown to express new or fetal antigens on their surface and theoretically these could act together with class I HLA antigens to attract cytotoxic T-cells.
- In immunosuppressed patients tumours are more common than in immunocompetent subjects; however, many of these are viral-associated cancers and it may be that the viruses are remaining unchecked rather than cancers no longer being repressed
- On balance there is still no convincing evidence that immune mechanisms are effective in the majority of cancers.

# 6

# Carcinogenesis

## Definitions

Carcinogen = substance, form of energy or organism capable of inducing a cancer (strictly this includes benign neoplasms also).

Mutagen = substance, form of energy or organism capable of inducing a mutation (a mutation may or may not produce a cancer but all cancers have some sort of mutation and all carcinogens are mutagens).

Mutation = an alteration in DNA from the usual sequence to a new sequence; this may produce no apparent effect or any of a wide range of diseases depending on its site (mutations are copied to every subsequent generation of cells but can only appear in subsequent individuals if they occur in the germ cells of the ovary or testis).

Oncogene = a sequence of DNA, usually a functional sequence, that by its non-physiological presence, relocation or mutation is capable of producing a cancer.

Cancer = malignant neoplasm.

Anti-oncogene = an oncogene that causes cancer by its absence.

Multistep hypothesis = it is thought that one mutation is generally not enough to produce cancer; several, occurring in the correct sequence, are probably needed.

Epidemiology = the study of the distribution of disease in populations (in both space and time).

Clone = a group of cells having the same genotype and phenotype and being derived from one progenitor cell.

Genotype = the genetic constitution of a cell or organism.

Phenotype = the physical expression of the genotype.

## Methods of investigating carcinogenesis

### Epidemiology

- If a disease occurs with a higher than expected frequency in a particular area or at a particular time, it may be possible to associate this with some other factor with the same distribution and identify a possible causal agent.

- This has been done with success for several cancers, for example hepatoma (hepatocellular carcinoma), which is commonly found in the presence of cirrhosis and rarely in its absence.
- The commonest cause of cirrhosis in the western world is alcohol; the commonest cause in the rest of the world is hepatitis B and mycotoxins (such as aflatoxin):
    (a) hepatitis B may be directly carcinogenic (the virus is incorporated into liver cell genomes) and aflatoxin causes specific point mutations in *p53*, while alcohol probably cause cirrhosis first (mycotoxins have been difficult to study since they occur in the same distribution as hepatitis B).
- *Lung cancer*: this shows a very close correlation with cigarette smoking, which is by far the most significant cause; other environmental factors such as pollution may be involved in some cases but tobacco is far more important:
    (a) the association is strongly dose related;
    (b) experimental evidence also clearly supports this.
- *Basal cell and squamous cell carcinoma*: these are commonest in elderly, fair-skinned people with chronic sun exposure:
    (a) manual outdoor occupations with high sun exposure are at high risk and this produces a secondary association with lower socio-economic status.
- *Malignant melanoma (melanocarcinoma)*: this occurs mainly in young, pale-skinned individuals with acute, severe, episodic sun exposure (usually holidays in high sun areas resulting in sunburn):
    (a) this produces secondary associations with higher socio-economic status and higher educational level;
    (a) a rare melanoma (lentigo maligna melanoma) occurs in the elderly in association with chronic sun exposure. Thus there are two incidence peaks for melanoma, pointing to two different aetiologies
- *Oesophageal carcinoma*: this shows a very specific distribution geographically (China and parts of Iran) but no firm evidence has yet emerged as to the nature of the carcinogen (dyes used in carpet making, dietary habits, opium, nitrosamines and human papilloma viruses have all been suggested) (*Figure 6.1*).

## Individual predisposition

- It is apparent that some diseases appear to run in families. This may be related to similar lifestyles and environmental factors, but in many cases it appears to be a true genetic tendency and some rare but striking 'cancer families' have been described.

- In most cases, particularly with the most common cancers, we do not have a clear idea of the mechanisms involved, but in some of the more obscure diseases the mechanisms have been well established.
- Although rare, these diseases are of great importance for the information that they give us about the normal function of the affected processes (so-called 'natural experiments'):

  (a) *xeroderma pigmentosum*: this is a rare disease in which children develop a range of cancers on the skin which are usually associated with old age;

    (i) although it is an heterogeneous disease with seven varieties the basic fault has been identified as a defect in DNA repair mechanism;

    (ii) this implies that ultraviolet (UV) light is damaging DNA in the skin of normal individuals at a considerable rate but in most people the damaged DNA is rapidly repaired with great fidelity;

    (iii) other conditions of this general sort include Bloom's syndrome, ataxia-telangiectasia and Fanconi's anaemia.

  (b) multiple endocrine neoplasia syndromes (MEN): there are three of these syndromes (variously classified) with a range of neoplasms occurring in endocrine organs; the mechanisms are obscure:

    (i) in many cases they seem to show a transition from hyperplasia to neoplasia.

  (c) *familial polyposis coli*: autosomal dominant disease with thousands of polyps and a 100% chance of developing colonic carcinoma if untreated by total colectomy:

    (i) the abnormality has been mapped to the long arm of chromosome 5 which is also found to bear a mutation in the common sporadic form of colonic carcinoma;

    (ii) this rare disease offers strong support to the theory that all colonic carcinomas begin as benign adenomatous polyps (adenoma–carcinoma sequence).

## Breast cancer

- There is a markedly increased risk of breast cancer in first-degree relatives of breast cancer patients.
- Very high rates of breast cancer in mice can be produced by selective breeding.

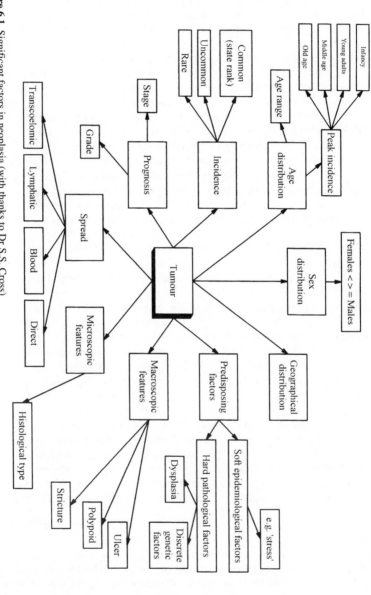

**Figure 6.1** Significant factors in neoplasia (with thanks to Dr S.S. Cross)

- A susceptibility gene has been found on chromosome 17q21 in many families with early breast cancer risk.

Nicholson R.I., McClelland R.A. and Gee J.M.W. (1995) Steroid hormone receptors and their clinical significance in cancer. *J. Clin. Pathol.*, **48**, 890–895.

## Occupational risk

Occupational risk is a form of epidemiological study which shows a risk associated with some carcinogen (usually chemical) in the workplace.

- *Scrotal cancer*: this is historically important since it was the first occupational cancer to be described fully (1777):
  - (a) it was described in chimney sweeps who had high and prolonged exposure to polycyclic aromatic hydrocarbons in soot;
  - (b) it is also described in machine tool workers exposed to lubricating oils;
  - (c) subsequent animal experimental demonstrations have supported this aetiology.
- *Mesothelioma*: workers in the building industry, ship construction and demolition were often exposed to high levels of asbestos dust as were the miners who mined it:
  - (a) the association between asbestos and mesothelioma was not apparent for some time, as the delay between exposure and the development of the tumour could be as long as 30 years;
  - (b) the wives of these workers also show a high incidence of mesothelioma as they were exposed to asbestos dust when washing clothing;
  - (c) the miners' families, were also heavily exposed if they lived close to the mineworks.
- *Bladder cancer*: workers in dye and rubber industries have a high risk of developing bladder cancer due to β-naphthylamine:
  - (a) even with careful protection, screening via urine cytology is necessary (together with cystoscopy if abnormalities are found) and compensation is routinely paid if such workers develop cancer as the association is so strong.
- *Carcinoma of the cervix*: although the great majority of cases are not associated with prostitution, this is an occupational risk amongst prostitutes since it is associated with multiple partners, early onset of intercourse and is associated with human papilloma virus infection:
  - (a) the acquired immuno deficiency syndrome (AIDS) risk is now so high that most prostitutes will insist on condoms and we may expect to see carcinoma of the cervix diminish in this high-risk group.

## Iatrogenic risk

Several medical interventions have been shown to produce cancer even though, at the time, they were thought to be entirely safe.

- *Arsenic*: this was used in a number of 'tonics' such as 'Parishes Food' and as an effective treatment for psoriasis in the form of 'Fowler's Solution'
    - (a) after long exposure and long delay such patients developed squamous carcinoma on non-sun-exposed skin and intestinal carcinoma.
- *Radiation*: this was used to shrink the thymus in young children who were thought to be suffering from thymic hyperplasia since the thymus was known to be atrophic in the adult; many of these children subsequently developed thyroid carcinoma.
- *Thorotrast*: this was used as a contrast medium for several years but has subsequently been shown to cause cholangiocarcinoma:
    - (a) thorotrast dioxide is an alpha particle emitter with a long half-life and is taken up by phagocytic cells and so lodged in the liver sinusoids.

# Classes of carcinogens

- Carcinogens are of many types: radiation; chemicals; unhealed or repeated trauma; and organisms.
- Added to this are the oncogenes, which are often just the results of mutations caused by a variety of mechanisms.

## Radiation

- Many forms of radiation from UV and ionizing radiation down to various subatomic particles will cause mutations.
- The shorter the wavelength, the higher the energy of the radiation. Cyclic structures such as the bases in DNA absorb energy of short wavelength and the molecules become energized with the resultant breaking of chemical bonds and the formation of new ones.
- If these are not repaired by the numerous repair processes, then they persist as mutations.
- Most of these mutations are lethal to the cell or cause no significant effect because they are in 'junk' DNA.

## Chemical carcinogens

- Many chemical carcinogens are not themselves active but are activated by body defence mechanisms.

- This occurs because many detoxification systems are stereotyped (such as mixed function oxidases) and remove reactive groups from molecules, usually resulting in a less active molecule but sometimes producing a more active species such as free radicals.
- There are species differences and guinea pigs lack the enzyme for the activation of acetylaminofluorene, which is therefore not carcinogenic in them although it is in most other species.
- Polycyclic aromatic hydrocarbons are the precursor substances responsible for skin cancer from tar derivatives; they are activated in the skin by aryl carbohydrate hydroxylase and cause cancers at that site.
- If they are absorbed systemically (as in cigarette smoke), they can cause cancers at distant sites such as the bladder as the enzyme is present in all tissues.
- Nitrosamines have been shown to produce cancer in animal models and bacterial action in the human gut can produce nitrosamines from nitrates and nitrites, which are commonly used as fertilizers and food additives, respectively.
- Numerous metals have been shown to be carcinogenic, mainly in industrial situations, these include: nickel; cadmium; cobalt; chromium; lead; and arsenic.

## Trauma

- There is clinical evidence that persistent trauma of various sorts, such as chronic ulceration, unstable fractures, chronic osteomyelitis and Paget's disease of bone, can lead to eventual malignancy; this seems to be related to the continued drive for cell replication in these conditions and may just be a statistical event due to the vast number of cell divisions occurring.
- Lymphangiosarcoma can arise in the chronically dilated lymphatic vessels following axillary clearance for breast cancer.
- *Schistosoma* eggs in the bladder are associated with squamous metaplasia and squamous carcinoma of the bladder, which is probably due to the chronic irritation associated with these eggs.
- *Chlonorchis sinensis* (Chinese liver fluke) lives in the bile ducts and can be associated with adenocarcinoma, presumably due to the long-term inflammation and irritation that it produces.

## Viral carcinogenesis

- Viruses are lengths of nucleic acid (DNA or RNA) that are obligate parasites which use a host cell's replicative machinery to reproduce themselves.

- During this process they may become incorporated into the host cell's DNA and in this site may produce a cancer.
- Examples of both DNA and RNA viruses are known to cause cancer in some animals but only one RNA virus has, as yet, been implicated in human cancers; this is human T-cell leukaemia virus type I (HTLV-I) related to the AIDS virus.
- An oncogenic virus uses the cell's replicative processes so there is selective advantage to the virus to induce host cell replication by activating genes for cell growth (growth factors and their receptors) and replication and for DNA synthesis; such unregulated growth may result in cancer.
- DNA viruses can enter the replication system directly but RNA viruses must first be copied as a DNA template which can then be used to synthesize more RNA virus. Such viruses contain a sequence for the enzyme reverse transcriptase which copies RNA as DNA.
- Relatively few human cancers are thought to be directly due to viruses and their main interest is that during evolution they seem to have picked up and carried DNA sequences from one cell to another; many of these sequences are what we recognize as oncogenes.
- Epstein–Barr virus (EBV; DNA herpes virus) is associated with a B-cell lymphoma seen in young children in endemic malarial areas of Africa, called Burkitt's lymphoma.
- The disease requires the virus and, probably, malarial infection for its expression. On its own the virus causes infectious mononucleosis.
- EBV is also associated with nasopharyngeal carcinoma in the Far East.
- Hepatitis-B virus is associated with cirrhosis of the liver and is probably directly oncogenic.
- The human papilloma virus is associated with benign skin tumours in experimental animals but may be associated with human carcinoma of the cervix.

Farrell P.J. and Tidy J. (1989) Viruses and human cancer. *Recent Adv. Histopathol.*, **14**, 23–41.
Herrington C.S. (1995) Human papillomaviruses and cervical neoplasia. II. Interactions of HPV with other factors. *J. Clin. Pathol.*, **48**, 1–6.

# Carcinogenesis

## Latency

- The causal event in carcinogenesis is usually followed by a variable, but lengthy, delay period.
- This latency is due in part to the fact that more than one event is required for cancer to develop (multistep theory) and partly to the

fact that it takes some time for the mutated cell to produce a clone of significant numbers to grow exponentially (the Gompertz sigmoid growth curve).

## Initiation

- The concept of *initiation* and *promotion* in relation to the generation of cancer comes mainly from experiments involving the production of skin tumours in mice, but some signs of these processes are also visible in human cancers ('field changes').
- Initiators cause mutations in cells but not full transformation to cancers; however, they predispose the cell to transformation by a promoter.
- Initiators vary widely in chemical structure but all are electrophilic or are converted to active electrophilic substances (electrophilic = having electron-deficient atoms and capable of reacting with electron-rich molecules such as nucleic acids and proteins).

## Promotion

- A promoter is a substance that will cause cancer in an initiated cell but not in a normal cell.
- Promoters are non-carcinogenic themselves unless they follow applications of initiators. They include: phorbol esters; hormones; phenols; and some drugs.

# Oncogenes and anti-oncogenes

## Oncogenes

- Several classes of oncogene have now been described (*Table 6.1*) but this does not preclude the future discovery of further oncogenes with radically different modes of action.
- There is a sequence of events controlling cell proliferation:
  (a) growth factor (GF) release;
  (b) binding to the extracellular domain of a receptor;
  (c) activation of the protein kinase associated with the intracellular domain of the receptor;
  (d) production of a second messenger which binds to the nucleus or DNA and modifies its expression.
- Oncogenes are the genes controlling each of these steps. It must be remembered that the oncogenes are the genes coding for active protein products which are the end effectors.

**Table 6.1 Classes of oncogenes**

| Class of oncogene | Example | Comments |
|---|---|---|
| Growth factor | *sis* coding for platelet-derived growth factor *int*-2 coding for a protein related to fibroblast growth factor | Growth factors in general cause cells to leave $G_0$ and to enter the cell cycle. *sis* appears to be involved in some brain tumours |
| Growth factor receptor | *erb* B coding for epidermal growth factor receptor | The *erb* family is often involved in breast cancer |
| Signal transducers | Tyrosine kinase | May be associated with growth factor receptors or attached to the cell membrane directly. *src* and the *ras* family are related to tyrosine kinase activities. The various *ras* family genes have been associated with a wide range of human tumours (bladder, breast, colorectum, lung, stomach) |
| Nuclear factors | *myc* has a DNA binding protein p62 | Unless *myc* is downregulated, the cell cannot leave the proliferative cycle. *jun* and *fos* are also nuclear binding factors but these regulate transcriptional activity of other genes. *myc* has been associated with many human cancers (breast, cervix, colorectum, prostate, stomach, lung, pancreas, testis) |

- There are several classes of genes that all interact in the production and prevention of tumours; these include:
  - (a) oncogenes;
  - (b) tumour suppresser genes;
  - (c) metastasis genes;
  - (d) apoptosis genes;
  - (e) DNA repair genes.

Royds J.A., Rees R.C. and Stephenson T.J. (1994) nm23 – a metastasis suppressor gene? *J. Pathol.*, **173**, 211–212.

## Anti-oncogenes

- In retinoblastoma it was proposed, and now demonstrated, that the tumour requires two mutational events for its expression.
- In inherited cases (about 40% of retinoblastoma cases) one *Rb* gene is lost or altered in the germline and expressed in every cell.

- As there are $10^7$ retinoblasts, the chance of a second mutation arising in a cell with one damaged or lost *Rb* gene is almost certain, consequently hereditary retinoblastoma is bilateral and occurs in almost all cases.
- Non-hereditary retinoblastoma cases are unilateral, since the chances of two mutational hits on the same cell are very low.
- The *Rb* gene product is a phosphoprotein involved in cell cycle regulation. The gene is expressed in all tissues and when it is unphosphorylated it stops entry of cells into the S phase.
- Phosphorylation inactivates the gene product and releases restraint on the cell cycle.
- Loss of or inactivation of *Rb* gene or product appears to be involved in numerous cancers.
- Several other candidate anti-oncogenes have been suggested but *Rb* is the best understood currently.

Cawkwell L. and Quirke P. (1994) Molecular genetics of cancer. *Recent Adv. Histopathol.*, **16**, 1–20.
Paul J. (1987) Oncogenesis. *Recent Adv. Histopathol.*, **13**, 13–31.

# 7

# Neoplasia

## Definitions

- Tumour = any neoplastic swelling (originally any swelling, neoplastic or not).
- Cancer = popular term used by the general public to indicate malignancy.
- Mitotic lesion = euphemism used by doctors in the presence of patients to mean malignant neoplasm.
- Hamartoma = embryological malformation; if it contains a mutation it will be different in type from those found in neoplasms. Usually containing more than one cell type they grow in proportion with the patient (neoplasms grow faster than the patient).
- Naevus = roughly equivalent to 'birthmark' and is a hamartoma. Naevocellular naevus consists of modified melanocytes which do not have dendrites.
- Mole = vague term; sometimes means birthmark, sometimes naevocellular naevus, sometimes a neoplasm of the placenta

## Classification

### Benign

- They do not invade (may locally infiltrate, i.e. pleomorphic adenoma of salivary gland). (Invasion = spread in continuity.)
- They will not metastasize. (Metastasis = spread in discontinuity.)
- Expansile growth.
- Slow growth.
- They are not expected to kill the patient.
- If they kill, they do so by pressure, erosion, etc., not metastasis.

### Malignant

- They have the potential to metastasize.
- They may invade locally.

- There is rapid growth.
- They have potential to kill the patient.

## Exceptions

- Basal cell carcinoma is very invasive but it does not metastasize. It is sometimes called 'locally malignant'.

## Features of malignancy

- Gross = unencapsulated. (May have a false capsule of compressed connective tissue but with strands of tumour spreading through, therefore unsafe to 'shell out', i.e. salivary gland tumours.)
- Invading adjacent tissue: may have areas of necrosis and haemorrhage.
- Histology: there is no such thing as 'malignant histology'; histology is only a morphological correlate of behaviour, it is not behaviour.
- Malignant features include:
  (a) disordered growth pattern;
  (b) variability in cell size (pleomorphism);
  (c) variability in nuclear size (pleomorphism);
  (d) high nuclear/cytoplasmic ratio;
  (e) multiple and bizarre nucleoli;
  (f) aberrant chromatin pattern;
  (g) increased number of mitoses;
  (h) aberrant mitoses.

# Nomenclature

Suffix -oma = benign neoplasm.
Suffix carcinoma = malignant epithelial neoplasm.
Suffix -sarcoma = malignant soft (or connective) tissue neoplasm.
Suffix -blastoma = tumour of immature or fetal type, i.e. retinoblastoma, nephroblastoma.
Teratoma = neoplasm of totipotential cells; can contain all germ lines, can be benign or malignant (terat = monster).

## Exceptions (misnomers)

Lymphoma: malignant, should be lymphosarcoma.
Hepatoma: malignant, should be hepatocellular carcinoma.
Melanoma: malignant, should be melanocarcinoma.

Most central nervous system (CNS) tumours are exceptions, i.e. glioma, glioblastoma, astrocytoma, etc.

## Macroscopic appearance

- *Papilloma*: fingerlike projections, often have a fibrovascular core. Papillary tumours often show calcification (thyroid). Papillae may protrude from epithelial surface (basal cell and squamous skin papillomas) or into cystic spaces (ovarian cystadenomas).
- *Cysts*: hollow structures lined by epithelium. Some old, large tumours may lose epithelial lining. Cysts may be neoplastic or mechanical (implantation dermoids of skin).
- *Multifocal*: multiple tumour masses showing no connection to each other. Difficult to explain in the case of benign tumours: possibility they are not benign and are metastases: possibility that areas of regression have isolated nodules; possibly not neoplastic but focal areas of hyperplasia (leiomyomas of uterus).
- *Mixed tumours*: tumours showing differentiation along more than one tissue line, usually epithelial and connective tissue (mixed tumour of salivary gland, mixed tumour of sweat gland, fibroadenoma of breast). Possibly epithelial component neoplastic and induces stromal component.
- *Collision tumours*: two different and independent tumours in contact.
- *Synchronous tumours*: two independent tumours arising at the same time.
- *Metachronous tumours*: two independent tumours arising sequentially.
- *Recurrence*: reappearance of a tumour following treatment (often misused to refer to a new tumour arising in a dysplastic field change).
- *Carcinoma-in-situ*: a lesion with all the cytological features of cancer but no evidence of invasion through the basement membrane (cf. cervical intra-epithelial neoplasia, CIN).

## Grading and staging

### Grading

- Pathological:
    - (a) malignant tumours can be graded; depends on various histological features, differs between tumours:
        - (i)   degree of differentiation (most epithelial tumours);

      (ii)  number of mitoses (differentiates leiomyomas from leiomyo-sarcomas);

     (iii)  abnormal mitoses, usually indicates malignancy (paradoxically the actual cell with an abnormal mitosis is very unlikely to produce viable daughter cells so that particular cell has no malignant potential).

- Grades: well, moderately or poorly differentiated. The rule of thumb is:
  - (a) well differentiated = difficult to be sure tumour is malignant;
  - (b) moderately differentiated = clearly malignant, tissue of origin still apparent;
  - (c) poorly differentiated = clearly malignant, difficult to determine tissue of origin but some clues;
  - (d) anaplastic = malignant neoplasm, could be anything.
- Nodal lymphoma grading is directly related to diagnostic category:
  - (a) any particular tumour usually a mixture of grades;
  - (b) prognosis depends on worst areas.
- Most pathology is based on small samples: cytology smallest; resections biggest; sampling errors can be high.
- One cannot *see* malignancy; appearance is only a morphological correlation which can be wrong.

### Prostate

- Grading: Gleeson histological grading pattern.

Bostwick D.G. (1994) Gleeson grading of prostatic needle biopsies. *Am. J. Surg. Path.*, **18**, 796–803.

### Bladder

- WHO grading system depends on:
  - (a) presence or absence of papillary pattern;
  - (b) thickness of epithelial layers;
  - (c) cytological atypia.
- Stage depends on:
  - (a) muscle invasion; often this cannot be determined on histology.

### Staging

- Mainly surgical, but many systems use pathological data.
- Different systems for different neoplasms (e.g. *Table 7.1*):
  - (a) TMN *t*opography, distant *m*etastasis, lymph *n*ode status.

Henson D.E. (1985) Staging for cancer: new developments and importance to pathology. *Arch. Pathol. Lab. Med.*, **109**, 13–16.

**Table 7.1 FIGO (International Federation of Gynaecology and Obstetrics) staging for ovarian tumours**

| Stage | | | Extent |
|---|---|---|---|
| I | | | Growth limited to the ovaries |
| | Ia | | Growth limited to one ovary; no ascites |
| | | 1 | No tumour on the external surface; capsule intact |
| | | 2 | Tumour on the external surface and/or capsule ruptured |
| | Ib | | Growth limited to both ovaries; no ascites |
| | | 1 | No tumour on the external surface; capsule intact |
| | | 2 | Tumour on the external surface and/or capsule(s) ruptured |
| | Ic | | Tumour either stage Ia or Ib but with ascites present or positive peritoneal washings |
| II | | | Growth involving one or both ovaries with pelvic extension |
| | IIa | | Extension and/or metastases to the uterus and/or tubes |
| | IIb | | Extension to other pelvic tissues |
| | IIc | | Tumour either stage IIa or IIb but with ascites or positive peritoneal washings |
| III | | | Growth involving one or both ovaries with intraperitoneal metastases outside the pelvis and/or positive retroperitoneal nodes. Tumour limited to the true pelvis with histologically proven malignant extension to small bowel or omentum |
| IV | | | Growth involving one or more ovaries with distant metastases. If pleural effusion is present there must be positive cytology to allot a case to stage IV. Parenchymal liver metastases equals stage IV |
| Special category | | | Unexplored cases which are thought to be ovarian carcinoma |

Scully R.E. (1982) *Tumors of the Ovary and Maldeveloped Gonads.* AFIP Fascicle 16, second series, Armed Forces Institute of Pathology, Washington DC.

## Colon and rectum

- Dukes: strictly only rectal but extrapolated to colorectal carcinoma generally (*Table 7.2*).
- Spread to other organs sometimes called stage D.

## Melanoma

- Melanoma prognosis is determined by the thickness of the tumour (Breslow) measured from granular layer of skin to the deepest malignant cell in mm (*Table 7.3*).
- Earlier Clark level still used because it is thought to be more biological as it refers to levels of invasion (*Table 7.4*). The best correlation with prognosis comes from Breslow thickness.

Mooi W.J. and Krausz T. (1992) *Biopsy Pathology of Melanocytic Disorders.* Chapman & Hall Medical, London.

**Table 7.2  Dukes' staging of rectal carcinoma (refers only to usual type adenocarcinoma, not squamous, melanoma, lymphoma, etc.)**

|  | Description | Stage | 5-year survival (%) |
|---|---|---|---|
| | Tumour confined to submucosa or muscle | Dukes A | 90+ |
| | Tumour spread through the muscle layer | Dukes B | 70 |
| | Any tumour involving lymph nodes | Dukes C | 35 |

# Metastasis

- Metastasis is tumour spread in discontinuity, as distinct from invasion which is spread in continuity.
- Tumours may metastasize across body cavities (i.e. thoracic or abdominal), by blood (haematogenous) or by lymph (lymphatic).
- Carcinomas tend to spread by lymphatic and haematogenous routes, sarcomas mostly by haematogenous routes.

**Table 7.3  Modified Breslow thickness values for malignant melanoma survival (Mooi & Krausz, 1992)**

| Maximal tumour thickness (mm) | 5-year survival (%) | 10-year survival (%) |
|---|---|---|
| < 0.76 | 97 | 94 |
| 0.76–1.49 | 88 | 82 |
| 1.5–2.49 | 77 | 63 |
| 2.5–3.99 | 71 | 61 |
| ≥ 4 | 47 | 40 |

**Table 7.4  Clark level for cutaneous melanoma survival**

| | Clark level | 5-year survival (%) | 10-year survival (%) |
|---|---|---|---|
| | I. All melanoma cells above the basement membrane | ≈ 100 | ≈ 100 |
| | II. Invasion of the papillary dermis | 96 | 93 |
| | III. Filling of the papillary dermis | 83 | 71 |
| | IV. Invasion of the reticular dermis | 71 | 59 |
| | V. Invasion of subcutaneous tissues | 52 | 36 |

- It is difficult to apply concepts of metastasis to lymphosarcomas since the nature of lymphoid cells is to circulate through the body. Circulating lymphomas are said to be in a leukaemic phase.
- Cellular abilities required for metastasis:
  (a) ability to invade locally;
  (b) ability to break off from main tumour mass;
  (c) ability to invade vessels;

    (d) ability to survive in blood or lymph;
    (e) ability to adhere to endothelium,
    (f)  ability to extravasate;
    (g) ability to grow in new site.

- These are not all simple mutations, nor all the same for different tumours, nor even the same for different clones within one tumour.
- Local invasion involves lysis of host tissue cells and degradation of extracellular matrix: tumours may induce fibroblast.
- Metalloproteinases, such as stromelysin 3, degrades extracellular matrix. Tumours may also produce metalloproteinases; fibroblasts or tumour cells may also produce inhibitors against the circulating inhibitors of metalloproteinases.
- Movement of tumour cells into lysed areas is stimulated by numerous factors derived from host or tumour cells and newly secreted basement membrane components.
- Cell adhesion properties are modified in tumours, allowing them to break off into the stroma – a process similar to loss of cell adhesion in culture. A family of proteins (cadherins) are responsible for cell adhesion and these have been shown to be modified in some tumours.
- The same mechanisms that promote stromal lysis and increased motility are thought to be responsible for vascular invasion.
- In the blood or lymph the tumour cells need to escape destruction by white cells and by antibodies attracted by the altered cell surface markers on the tumour cells; in relation to this there is evidence of loss of class I histocompatibility antigens on the cell surface of some tumours cells.
- Tiny clumps of cells are destroyed by turbulence and present large surface areas for attack by the immune system. Larger clumps (possibly protected by clotting on their surface) survive better.
- Arrest of circulating tumour clumps is mediated by integrins:
    (a) tumour cells also express the homing molecules (such as CD44) found on lymphocytes which enables them to locate specific tissues in the body.
- Most tumour clumps are killed when they arrest in the circulation, but those that escape the blood vessels are thought to do so by mechanisms similar to those that permit entry into vessels.
- In the new tissue site the tumour cells can produce autocrine growth factors and develop the ability to respond to local paracrine growth factors in order to grow there.
- Once established in the new site many tumours produce angiogenesis factors to promote new vessels for nutrition, and substances such as fibroblast growth factor and transforming growth factor to produce a supporting stroma.

- The genetic control of metastasis remains poorly understood but the metastasis suppresser gene *nm23* has been shown to be significantly reduced in a number of metastatic tumours.

Vile R.G. and Hart I.R. (1995) The molecular basis of metastasis. *Prog. Pathol.*, **1**, 133–150.

# Prognosis

Prognosis depends upon:
- type of tumour (epithelial, soft tissue origin, etc.);
- stage;
- grade;
- surface receptors (steroid receptors in breast cancer);
- oncogene and tumour suppressor gene expression;
- sensitivity to treatment modalities, including drug resistance;
- age of patient;
- coexisting disease;
- immune status and human leukocyte antigen (HLA) type;
- nutritional status;
- individual biological variation.

Underwood J.C.E. (1992) Prognostic indices in epithelial neoplasms. *Recent Adv. Histopathol.*, **15**, 17–36.

# Screening

Screening should be directed at the asymptomatic population at risk and must be:
- for a relatively common disease (gastric carcinoma in Japan but not UK);
- cheaper than treatment;
- acceptable to patients;
- highly accurate (low false-positive and -negative rates);
- accompanied by effective and acceptable therapy.

## Cervical screening

- Exfoliative cytology from asymptomatic women.
- Difficulty in determining cancer-in-situ led to the classification of Cervical Intraepithelial Neoplasia (CIN) grades I–III depending on thickness of change.

## CIN (cervical intraepithelial neoplasia)

### Definitions

CIN1 = undifferentiated neoplastic cells occupying no more than the lower one-third of the epithelium.

CIN2 = undifferentiated neoplastic cells occupying up to two-thirds vertically of the lower epithelium.

CIN3 = undifferentiated neoplastic cells occupying more than the vertical two-thirds of the lower epithelium.

- This is a related concept to carcinoma-in-situ but avoids the paradox of a malignant 'carcinoma' with no metastatic potential and permits comparison with the cytology gradings. Usually graded CIN1, 2 or 3 on the basis of the thickness of the lesion, which commonly equates with mild, moderate and severe dysplasia respectively.
- The lateral transition between normal and neoplastic may be very sharp and is called Schiller's line; sometimes the grading is subtle merging normal/CIN1/CIN2/CIN3.
- Severe change leads to biopsy and further surgery, if needed, correlates well with cytology.
- Screening programme has led to significant decrease in deaths from cervical cancer.

## Breast screening

- Screening is mammographic and supported by clinical examination and cytology of suspicious masses; this forms the triple approach.
- The age group at highest risk, 50–64 years, are screened in the UK.

### Grade

This is based on:
- tubule formation;
- nuclear pleomorphism;
- number of mitoses.
- Together these give the modified Bloom & Richardson grading which, together with node status and size of the tumour, is used to calculate the 'Nottingham Prognostic Index' Page and Anderson, 1987).

### Stage

- This is calculated on:

(a) stage I = node negative;
(b) stage II = low axillary node positive;
(c) stage III = high axillary or internal mammary node positive.

- The 'Nottingham Prognostic Index' correlates well with survival and can be used for counselling patients.

Page D.L. and Anderson T.J. (eds) (1987) *Diagnostic Histopathology of the Breast.* Churchill Livingstone, Edinburgh.

# 8

# Disorders of metabolism

## Accumulations

### Atheroma

- Atheroma is variously classified as a degenerative disease, a consequence of lifestyle and an ageing phenomenon but it is characterized by an accumulation of material in blood vessel walls causing atherosclerosis, which is the commonest form of 'hardening of the arteries' (arteriosclerosis).
- The incidence of atheroma increases with age and is therefore more common in the elderly.
- It is rare in young adults and very rare in children:
  (a) exceptions include the hypercholesterolaemias and progerias; patients in both of these groups often dying young from atheroma-associated diseases.

### *Predisposing factors in atheroma*

- Western lifestyle especially diet and sedentary occupation.
- Smoking.
- Diabetes mellitus.
- Positive family history.
- Obesity.
- Male sex.
- Increasing age.
- Oral contraception.
- 'Stress' (a popular idea, but lacking any formal proof).

### *Pathogenesis*

- The current view is termed the 'response to injury hypothesis'. It combines the elements of two previous theories: (a) infusion of blood proteins and lipids into intimal cells and (b) organization and repetitive growth of thrombi into plaques.

- It now seems that various modes of injury to the intima can initiate plaque formation.
- Loss of endothelium allows circulating monocytes and platelets to adhere to the damaged wall.
- These then enter the intima (presumably under the influence of monocyte chemotactic protein-1 (MCP-1) and macrophage colony stimulating factor (MCSF)) and take up lipids to form foamy macrophages.
- Foamy macrophages (foam cells) are capable of taking up oxidized low density liproteins (LDL) at very high rates, whereas untransformed macrophage LDL receptor is insensitive to these molecules which are produced in large amounts in the damaged vessel.
- The fatty streaks which are thought to be atheroma precursors in the vessel wall consist mainly of foam cells.
- The foam cells also secrete a number of growth factors (platelet-derived growth factor (PDGF), fibroblast growth factor (FGF), transforming growth factor beta (TGF-$\beta$)) capable of attracting in other cells such as platelets and lymphocytes.
- Smooth muscle cells, probably attracted in from the media, proliferate and are capable of accumulating large amounts of cholesterol, which is why there is such a strong association of atheroma with hypercholesterolaemia and fatty diets.
- The bulging plaque protrudes into the lumen causing turbulence in the blood flow and contributing to a tendency to thrombus formation because of pre-existing intimal damage and further damage caused by the turbulence.
- Hypertension may aggravate the problem by forcing lipids and proteins through the wall.
- The plaques commonly calcify and the major elastic arteries such as the aorta lose their elasticity.
- The increased pressures develop causing dilatation of the vessel (aneurysm) and these may eventually leak or rupture.
- In other cases the weakened intima may tear and allow blood to track in, producing a dissection.
- Not all aneurysms are associated with atheroma. Other causes of aneurysms include:
  (a) false aneurysm due to the walled-off blood from a ruptured vessel – the wall consists of fibrosis and other connective tissue;
  (b) arteriovenous aneurysm where a connection is established due to trauma or other damage; this can sometimes occur due to aortic atheroma eroding into the vena cava causing symptoms of leaking aortic aneurysm which cannot be detected at operation (a clue to this is a spongy pulsatile liver which can be seen at operation);

(c) dissections associated with collagen weakness (Marfan's syndrome, pregnancy, severe hypertension particularly in Afro-Americans);

(d) syphilitic aneurysms due to inflammation of the aortic vasa vasora;

(e) aneurysms are also classified on their shape, independent of their aetiology, i.e. saccular, fusiform.

• Since atheroma predisposes to thrombosis it often underlies devastating events such as coronary artery thrombosis and cerebro-vascular accidents (CVA) and transient ischaemic attacks (TIA)

Ernst C.B. (1993) Abdominal aortic aneurysm. *N. Engl. J. Med.*, **328**, 1167–1172.

Cigarroa J.E., Isselbacher E.M., DeSanctis R.W. and Eagle K.A. (1993) Diagnostic imaging in the evaluation of suspected aortic dissection. Old standards and new directions. *N. Engl. J. Med.*, **328**, 35–43.

Ferns G.A.A. and Woolaghan E. (1995) Recent insights into the mechanisms of iatrogenic arteriosclerosis. *J. Pathol.*, **176**, 331–332.

## Amyloidosis

• Many processes of cell damage generate large amounts of meta-bolically active proteins (enzymes, hormones, shock proteins).

• These proteins are rendered inert by being transformed into antiparallel β-pleated sheets.

• They are deposited extracellularly, often around blood vessels.

• The human has no enzymes for these protein configurations so they accumulate.

• Clinical symptoms are due to amyloid accumulation.

• The various amyloids are chemically different but physically similar.

• A characteristic ring glycoprotein (substance P) is deposited on amyloid.

• Many amyloids are known but the two commonest consist of immunoglobulin light chains (amyloid light chain (AL)) and a protein produced in the liver (amyloid-associated protein (AA)), which is associated with chronic inflammation (rheumatoid disease, osteomyelitis) and is related to acute-phase proteins.

• Some endocrine tumours produce excess protein hormone which may be converted to amyloid (e.g. medullary carcinoma of the thyroid).

• Amyloid also occurs in the brain in association with Alzheimer plaques and in various other ageing tissues.

Tan S.Y. and Pepys M.B. (1994) Amyloidosis. *Histopathology*, **25**, 403–414.

Looi L.M. (1993) Amyloids and tactoids. *J. Pathol.*, **170**, 417–418.

Cornwell III G.G., Johnson K.H. and Westermark P. (1995) The age related amyloids: a growing family of unique biochemical substances. *J. Clin. Pathol.*, **48**, 984–989.

## Lipofuscin

- Heterogeneous collection of metabolic end-products which accumulate in ageing cells.
- These occur at least partly due to peroxidation of membranes.
- They are more a marker of ageing than a cause.
- Lipofuscin accumulates rapidly in the central nervous system (CNS) in Batten's syndrome, with blindness and mental deterioration.

## Calcification

- Calcium metabolism is controlled by a balance between the active form of vitamin D (1,25-dihydroxyvitamin D) and parathyroid hormone (PTH); the role of calcitonin remains obscure.
- Heterotopic calcification = calcification occurring at abnormal sites.
- Dystrophic calcification = calcification occurring at abnormal tissues. It occurs in: the absence of hypercalcaemia; established atheroma; ageing, damaged or congenitally abnormal heart valves; papillary carcinomas as psammoma bodies (thyroid, ovary); tuberculous lesions; commonly in breast cancer (mammographic screening); may result in heterotopic bone formation; since cell death involves influx of calcium a single cell can often be the nidus for calcium accretion.
- Metastatic calcification = calcification occurring in otherwise normal tissues. It appears to begin in mitochondria; occurs in the presence of hypercalcaemia of any cause (hyperparathyroidism, high vitamin D levels, sarcoidosis, hyperthyroidism, Addison's disease, increased bone catabolism); affects mainly vessels, kidneys, lungs and gastric mucosa.
- Acute hypercalcaemia results in fits, vomiting and polyuria; hypocalcaemia results in tetany.

## Gout

- Uric acid results from DNA breakdown and is excreted by the kidney.
- High intake, low excretion, genetics, increased DNA breakdown (i.e. chemotherapy, radiotherapy) results in hyperuricaemia and precipitation in skin (tophi), kidneys (calculi), and joints (synovitis and arthritis).
- Commoner in males; there is often a family history. It is related to a high meat and high alcohol diet. The site of predilection is the first metatarsophalangeal joint.

## Other crystals

- Many crystals are optically active and will change the direction of polarized light, sometimes in such a specific way as to be diagnostic; this is carried out using polarizing filters.
- Cholesterol crystals:
  (a) may deposit in tissues when there is excess breakdown of fats or lipid-rich membranes;
  (b) most commonly seen in atherosclerosis;
  (c) the crystals are long and pointed at the ends;
  (d) since they are soluble in the solvents used in histology they appear as crystal-shaped holes in the sections;
  (e) they can be demonstrated using frozen sections and lipid stains.
- Calcium pyrophosphate:
  (a) causes pseudo-gout;
  (b) there is a sporadic hereditary type and a secondary type associated with joint damage, hyperparathyroidism and diabetes mellitus;
  (c) rectangular, birefringent crystals form in cartilage and then rupture into joint spaces;
  (d) the mechanism of the disease is unknown.
- Other accumulations of crystals include:
  (a) calcium oxalate in oxalosis;
  (b) cystine in cystinosis;
  (c) tyrosine in tyrosinosis.
- Exogenous crystals include:
  (a) barium sulphate;
  (b) asbestos;
  (c) silica;
  (d) starch;
  (e) talc.

## Hyaline change

- This is a histological term referring to a glassy appearance of cells or matrix arising for a variety of reasons.

## Pigments

- Any substance that causes a change in tissue colour is a pigment.
- Pigments may be *endogenous* or *exogenous* in origin.
- They may have pathological effects or they may be inert indicators of some pathological process.
- *Endogenous pigments* are coloured materials normally present in metabolism but occurring in excess amounts or unusual places.

## Black

- Melanin: condensation product of dopamine made in melanocytes in the skin and retina but occurring incidentally in dopaminergic areas of the brain (substantia nigra). Increased amounts occur in the skin on exposure to ultraviolet (UV) light. There are small foci in freckles (ephilis), increased numbers of melanocytes in lentigo, moles and melanomas. They may stain tissues (melanism) or be excreted in large amounts in the urine in widespread metastatic melanoma (melanuria). Melanin has no direct harmful effect.
- Pigmentary deficiency: albinism is a group of diseases where melanin synthesis is deficient; vitiligo is an auto-immune disease that destroys melanocytes; some dark-skinned people lighten their skin with various chemicals.
- Carbon: in lungs and thoracic lymph nodes due to exposure to tobacco, coal dust (anthracosis in miners), atmospheric pollution:
  (a) in skin from coalface work (miners), amateur tattoos.
- Formalin can produce artefactual black pigment in histology.
- Malaria pigment is black.
- Polymerized homogentisic acid in alkaptonuria causes ochronosis when it binds to cartilage; it can be seen in ears and can cause arthritis in joints. Urine turns black on standing; sweat may be black.
- Silver binds to basement membranes in argyria, which is usually caused by industrial exposure.

## Brown

- Melanosis coli: nothing to do with melanin, it is a coloration of the large intestine due to anthracene laxative abuse (variously said to be anthracene pigment, lipofuscin and apoptotic bodies).
- Haemosiderin: breakdown product of haemoglobin, seen in resolving haematomas (these undergo numerous colour changes including green and yellow).
- Raised circulating bile pigments bind to elastin and are most visible in the sclera and skin (jaundice); they also colour elastic blood vessels strongly and accumulate in the liver (cholestasis).
- Lipofuscin (ageing pigment) is a golden-brown intracellular pigment which is a complex mixture of peroxidized lipids probably of membrane origin. It is responsible for 'brown atrophy', which is a combination of senile involution of organs and the accumulation of lipofuscin.
- Copper deposition in the corneal limbus (Kayser–Fleischer rings) and lilac fingernails occur in hepatolenticular degeneration (Wilson's disease) with cirrhosis and basal ganglia damage mediated by free radical damage.

### Blue

- Cyanosis is due to poor oxygenation of tissues and may be peripheral, as in simple coldness, or central, due to poor oxygenation of blood.
- A blue naevus is a deep, melanocytic naevus which appears blue due to the Tyndall effect (scattering of light, preferentially short wavelength, by colloidal-sized molecules, the same mechanism that makes the sky blue).

### Other colours

- Professional tattoos use many colours and some subjects show allergies or photosensitivity reactions. The pigment is located in the dermis and removal of the epidermis will not affect the tattoo.
- Bruises, haematomas, *erythema ab igne* and chronic venous stasis all have some extravasation of blood and produce the same range of brown/green/yellow pigmentation as the haemoglobin is metabolized.

# Hormonal

## Diabetes

### Definitions

- Diabetes = excess urine output.
- Mellitus = the urine contains sugar.
- Insipidus = the urine does not contain sugar.

### Diabetes insipidus

- Diabetes insipidus is a failure in pituitary antidiuretic hormone (ADH) or a lack of renal sensitivity to ADH.

### Primary diabetes mellitus

- This includes insulin-dependent diabetes (IDDM), also called type I, and non-insulin-dependent diabetes mellitus (NIDDM), also called type II or maturity-onset diabetes mellitus.
- NIDDM includes non-obese NIDDM, obese NIDDM and maturity-onset NIDDM of the young.

## Aetiology

- *IDDM*: a failure to produce active insulin from islets of Langerhans in the pancreas; presents in childhood; high titres of Coxsackie B and mumps virus; early lesions show lymphocytic infiltrate suggesting autoimmune cause; associated with HLA-DR4 particularly together with HLA-B8 and HLA-D3; thought to be caused by viral infection in susceptible individuals triggering autoimmune destruction of islets.

Atkinson M.A. and Maclaren N.K. (1994) The pathogenesis of insulin-dependent diabetes mellitus. *N. Engl. J. Med.*, **331**, 1428–1436.

- *NIDDM*: a failure of target tissues to respond to normal levels of insulin; presents in the middle-aged, generally obese patient. There is a strong genetic element (nearly 100% identical twin concordance).

### Secondary diabetes mellitus

- This involves high levels of hormones which counteract insulin from tumours or other diseases, i.e. glucagonoma, Cushing's syndrome, phaeochromocytoma and acromegaly.
- It includes destruction of the pancreas from any cause, i.e. acute or chronic pancreatitis, haemochromatosis.

### Effects of diabetes mellitus

- Diabetes mellitus is a multisystem disease whose effects are mainly due to small vessel damage (microangiopathy) and accelerated atheroma formation.
- Complications include:
  - (a) glomerular damage leading to nephrotic syndrome and renal failure;
  - (b) increased risk of infection;
  - (c) poor wound healing;
  - (d) cataracts;
  - (e) ketoacidosis;
  - (f) hyperosmolar diabetic coma;
  - (g) insulin therapy-related hypoglycaemia.

## Other hormone states

- Hormonal diseases may be due to excess or deficiency.
- They may be due to overactivity or underactivity of the gland itself.

- They may be due to abnormalities in the control of the gland (hypothalamic or pituitary abnormalities may affect the production of hormones from target endocrine organs).
- Hormonal states due to alterations in trophic hormones:
  - (a) prolactinoma: causes galactorrhoea and menstrual disturbances;
  - (b) growth hormone (GH): causes gigantism in children or acromegaly in adults;
  - (c) thyroid stimulating hormone (TSH): causes hyperthyroidism;
  - (d) *a*mine content and/or *p*recursor *u*ptake and *d*ecarboxylation tumours (APUD) may produce a variety of hormones including active amines (serotonin) or proteins. The term APUD refers to the test used to recognize the tissue, not to the type of hormone produced (it is not a good term but still used). Ectopic hormone-producing tumours of many organs occur; lung tumours can produce many peptide and amine hormones;
  - (e) carcinoids: produce serotonin. Those in the gut do not produce enough hormone to cause carcinoid syndrome (flushing, cardiac dysrhythmia, pulmonary valve stenosis, diarrhoea) until they metastasize to the liver;
  - (f) insulinoma and glucagonoma: tumours of islet cells producing insulin or glucagon repectively.
- Gastrinoma arise in the pancreas (90%) or duodenum (10%). They produce gastrin and Zollinger–Ellison syndrome (peptic ulcer disease, gastric hypersecretion, pancreatic islet cell tumour).
- Phaeochromocytoma is a rare tumour of the adrenal medulla (15% arise in extra-adrenal paraganglia). It produces catecholamine-induced hypertension which can be cured surgically. It may be associated with a variety of multiple endocrine neoplasia (MEN) syndromes.
- Autoimmune hormonal states:
  - (a) autoimmune states may be general or organ-specific; hormonal ones are organ-specific as they are related to specific endocrine organs;
  - (b) organ-specific autoimmune states tend to occur together;
  - (c) they are more common in females;
  - (d) they are often associated with specific HLA types;
  - (e) they may stimulate or suppress endocrine glands;
  - (f) Graves' thyroiditis is hyperthyroidism produced by IgG autoantibodies, which bind to epithelial cells of the thyroid and mimic the action of TSH;
  - (g) Hashimoto's thyroiditis is hypothyroidism (sometimes following a brief phase of hyperthyroidism as hormones are released from damaged cells) produced by autoimmune destruction of thyroid cells.

# Nutrition

## Surgical nutrition

- Surgery, in common with any other traumatic experience, has wide metabolic consequences.
- The postsurgical state has been divided into four:
  - (a) the catabolic phase;
  - (b) the turning point phase;
  - (c) the restitution of lean body mass phase;
  - (d) and the fat gain phase.
- These phases are modified by many factors including the pre-operative nutritional state of the patient, which can affect surgical outcome greatly.
- Careful nutritional preparation of the patient is needed for the successful outcome of surgery, particularly in the elderly.
- The extent of injury and the presence or absence of infection also affect the length of the catabolic phase.
- A prolonged or severe catabolic phase can have a significant mortality.
- The shortest term cellular energy store is ATP, which is used up in seconds.
- Liver glycogen may last a few hours but its utilization overlaps with the next energy source, which is lipid and then protein.
- This produces a series of metabolic problems including ketosis and eventual loss of proteins from body mass, plasma proteins, immunoglobulins, wound repair processes and metabolic substances, such as clotting factors and enzymes generally.
- Other factors affect nutritional status, including loss of appetite due to pain and to the side-effects of drugs.
- Balanced parenteral nutrition is essential for all patients who may be expected to have any significant or prolonged reduction in food intake by the oral route.
- The various nutritional routes include:
  - (a) oral;
  - (b) enteric tube feeding;
  - (c) intravenous supplements;
  - (d) total parenteral nutrition.
- Patients needing extra nutritional care include:
  - (a) elderly, surgical patients;
  - (b) patients with burns;
  - (c) extensive trauma cases;
  - (d) head injuries;
  - (e) cancer patients.

## Effects of alcohol

- Ethyl alcohol is the main ingredient of alcoholic drinks.
- Methyl alcohol is sometimes used to make non-potable alcohol preparations undrinkable, although people still drink them.
- Pure methyl alcohol can cause permanent blindness in doses as small as 5 ml.
- Ethyl alcohol is an intoxicant and can be lethal in acute overdose (acute alcohol poisoning must be reported to the Coroner; chronic alcohol poisoning no longer has to be referred).
- Lethal blood levels can be very variable but there is significant risk above 300 mg/dl.
- Levels several times this have been found in chronic alcohol abusers who have, nevertheless, survived.
- Ethyl alcohol (ethanol), or perhaps its metabolites such as acetaldehyde, has direct effects on mitochondria and microsomes.
- A small proportion of alcohol is metabolized by gastric mucosal alcohol dehydrogenase but most enters the bloodstream. The majority is metabolized in the liver by three main pathways:
  - (a) hepatic alcohol dehydrogenase is the main one, resulting in the production of acetaldehyde which is then converted by aldehyde dehydrogenase to acetate;
  - (b) P-450 is an inducible liver enzyme that is upregulated to deal with a wide range of ingested toxins; in the case of alcohol it again produces acetaldehyde;
  - (c) a small amount is metabolized by peroxisomal catalase.
- These processes result in an increased NADH:NAD ratio which inhibits the oxidation of fatty acids causing them to accumulate in the hepatocytes and leading to the typical alcoholic fatty liver.

### Other acute effects of alcohol

The other acute effects of alcohol are mostly psychosocial, which is, of course, why people drink it:
- mood change is prominent;
- loss of inhibition;
- impairment of judgement;
- aggression.

### Chronic effects of alcohol

The chronic effects also involve behavioural changes but also more long-lasting physical damage:
- liver disease is a prominent feature of chronic alcohol use;
- it is said that five large whiskies, five pints of beer or a bottle of wine a day are hepatotoxic over a period of about 3–5 years in about one-

third of alcoholics and about one-third of these will progress to develop cirrhosis;

- women are more susceptible than men;
- alcoholic hepatitis commonly develops on fatty liver disease and shows ballooning and necrosis of hepatocytes together with a neutrophil infiltrate around hepatic veins;
- fibrillary Mallory's hyalin accumulates in cells, together with giant mitochondria;
- fibrosis occurs progressively and eventually becomes cirrhosis (nodules of regenerating liver drowning in a sea of fibrosis);
- this micronodular cirrhosis progresses and an element of macronodular cirrhosis may also occur, but the important feature is the disruption of the liver vasculature;
- this disruption results in systemic venous pressure back into the portal system with eventual distension and formation of oesophageal varices and their rupture;
- eventually liver failure supervenes and patients may develop hepatic encephalopathy due to their inability to metabolize toxins;
- bleeding disorders also develop because of the failure to produce clotting factors;
- cerebral pathology may occur secondarily to the dietary deficiency of thiamine (vitamin $B_1$) and result in Wernicke–Korsakoff syndrome with short-term memory loss and various neurological features;
- pancreatitis is a common complication of alcoholism and may be acute or chronic;
- alcohol causes acute pancreatitis by inducing pancreatic excretory duct inflammation with resultant pancreatic necrosis;
- this may progress to chronic pancreatitis due to progressive fibrosis;
- on the plus side, small regular amounts of alcohol protect against myocardial disease.

Heys S.D., Park K.G., Garlick P.J. and Eremin O. (1992) Nutrition and malignant disease: implications for surgical practice. *Br. J. Surg.*, **79**, 614–623.
Steer M.L., Waxman I. and Freedman S. (1995) Chronic pancreatitis. *N. Engl. J. Med.*, **332**, 1482–1490.
Steinberg W. and Tenner S. (1994) Acute pancreatitis. *N. Engl. J. Med.*, **330**, 1198–1210.

# Water and electrolyte balance

Water and electrolyte homeostasis is controlled by several hormones.

## Antidiuretic hormone (ADH)

- Physiology: causes kidneys to resorb water, lowering urine output. Osmoreceptors in the hypothalamus detect lowered solute to water ratio and lower ADH secretion by the posterior pituitary.

- Pathology: some tumours (particularly lung) can secrete ADH. ADH can produce hypertension by causing constriction of arterioles (ADH is also known as vasopressin). Damage to the posterior pituitary or hypothalamus can result in lowered ADH secretion and diabetes insipidus. Alcohol inhibits ADH and causes relative dehydration (hangover).

## Aldosterone

- Physiology: mineralocorticoid secreted by adrenal cortex acts on renal tubular cells to resorb $Na^+$ and increase loss of $K^+$, water, $Cl^-$ and $HCO_3^-$ follow $Na^+$. Aldosterone also removes $H^+$ from the blood and helps to control pH. Decrease in blood volume causes release of renin from juxtoglomerular cells of kidney; renin converts inactive plasma angiotensinogen (produced by liver cells) to angiotensin I. Plasma angiotensin I is converted to angiotensin II by angiotensin-converting enzyme in the lungs. Angiotensin II stimulates the adrenal cortex to release aldosterone, and is also a powerful vasoconstrictor that helps to increase blood pressure.
- Pathology: tumours of the zona glomerulosa of the adrenal can cause hyperaldosteronism.

## Atrial natriuretic peptide

- Atrial cardiac fibres release atrial naturetic peptide when stretched and this hormone causes $Na^+$ and water loss and vasodilatation lowering blood pressure.

## Water loss

Water loss is a serious problem in:
- vomiting and diarrhoea;
- extensive burns;
- blistering diseases;
- excessive sweating (fever, hot climates, exercise);
- diabetes insipidus and nephrogenic diabetes insipidus;
- diuresis (IDDM or iatrogenic).

# Acid base balance (acid base homeostasis)

- General body metabolism functions best at about pH 7.4.
- Many enzymes have pH maxima at this level.

- Enzymes that function in an acid milieu have acid pH optima (stomach enzymes, lysosomal enzymes).
- The tendency of metabolism is towards acidosis ($CO_2$ from respiration, lactic acid from glycolysis and fatty acids from lipolysis), which is recognized by receptors (carotid bodies, aortic arch receptors and the brain medulla).
- Because metabolism leads to acid production, acidosis is the more common problem.
- Buffers counteract this (mainly bicarbonate and proteins) to some extent but the main control is by respiratory loss of $CO_2$, renal excretion of $H^+$, metabolism of lactate and fatty acids and production of bicarbonate.
- There are four main types of imbalance (*Tables 8.1* and *8.2*):
  (a) respiratory acidosis;
  (b) respiratory alkalosis;
  (c) metabolic acidosis;
  (d) metabolic alkalosis.

Bilezikian J.P. (1992) Management of acute hypercalcemia. *N. Engl. J. Med.*, **326**, 1196–1203.


# Gallstones (cholelithiasis)

- Gallstones are solidifications of the contents of bile; they occur almost exclusively in the gallbladder.
- In the West about 80% of stones contain more than 50% cholesterol with an admixture of other bile components.
- Pigment stones occur in the presence of haemolytic anaemias and are more common where the frequency of these is high.
- Factors associated with mixed stones and cholesterol stones are:
  (a) age;
  (b) female sex;
  (c) oral contraceptives;
  (d) pregnancy;
  (e) obesity;
  (f) rapid weight loss;
  (g) bile stasis and infection;
  (h) metabolic disorders of bile metabolism (*Figure 8.1*);
  (i) diabetes mellitus;
  (j) hypercholesterolaemia.
- Factors associated with pigment stones are:
  (a) haemolytic anaemias;
  (b) gallbladder infection.

**Table 8.1 Acidosis**

| Types of acidosis | Causative condition | pH | $Pa_{CO_2}$ | $HCO_3^-$ | Response |
|---|---|---|---|---|---|
| 1. Hydrogen ion excess with normal homeostasis | | N-↓ | N-↓ | ↓ | $HCO_3^-$ resorption and regeneration by kidney |
| (a) Ketoacidosis | (i) Diabetes mellitus | N-↓ | N-↓ | ↓ | |
| | (ii) Starvation or tissue damage | N-↓ | N-↓ | ↓ | |
| (b) Absolute hypoxia | Usually due to poor blood supply or shock (lactic acidosis) | N-↓ | N-↓ | ↓ | |
| (c) Relative hypoxia | (i) Muscular exercise (physiological) | N-↓ | N-↓ | ↓ | |
| | (ii) Starvation | N-↓ | N-↓ | ↓ | |
| (d) Excessive hydrogen ion intake | Usually iatrogenic | N-↓ | N-↓ | ↓ | |
| 2. Failure of homeostasis | | ↓ | ↓ | ↓ | pH can be normalized by hyperventilation, which can also further decrease $Pa_{CO_2}$ |
| (a) Failure of kidney to secrete hydrogen ions | (i) General renal failure | ↓ | ↓ | ↓ | |
| | (ii) Tubular failure/acidosis | ↓ | ↓ | ↓ | |
| | (iii) Low glomerular filtration rate | ↓ | ↓ | ↓ | |
| (b) Retention of $CO_2$ | (i) Acute respiratory failure | ↓ | ↑ | N-↑ | $CO_2$ diffuses into erythrocytes and is buffered by haemoglobin. Plasma production of $HCO_3^-$ is driven by ↑ $CO_2$ |
| | (ii) Chronic respiratory failure | N-↓ | ↑ | ↑ | Increased $Pa_{CO_2}$ may drive $HCO_3^-$ regeneration enough to correct $CO_2$ levels |
| 3. Relative $H^+$ excess in $HCO_3^-$ depletion | | ↓ | ↓ | ↓ | $H^+$ secretion in urine and $HCO_3^-$ reabsorbtion and regeneration |
| (a) Loss of intestinal $HCO_3^-$ | Fistulae, severe diarrhoea | ↓ | ↓ | ↓ | |
| (b) Transplantation of ureters into colon | Resorption of $Cl^-$ for $HCO_3^-$ plus bacterial conversion of urea to ammonia | ↓ | ↓ | ↓ | |

**Table 8.2  Alkalosis**

| Types of alkalosis | Causative condition | pH | $Pa_{CO_2}$ | $HCO_3^-$ | Response |
|---|---|---|---|---|---|
| 1. Alkalosis with normal homeostasis | Due to an effective loss of $H^+$ | ↑ | N | ↑ | Vomiting from stomach loses $H^+$ but from duodenum loses $HCO_3^-$, so if both occur they may be balanced |
| (a) Ingestion of large amounts of soluble base | Milk alkali syndrome | ↑ | N | ↑ | |
| (b) Loss of unbuffered $H^+$ | Pyloric stenosis | ↑ | N | ↑ | |
| (c) $K^+$ depletion | Vomiting causes extracellular alkalosis with intracellular acidosis | ↑ | N | ↑ | |
| 2. Alkalosis due to abnormal homeostasis | Always due to over-breathing | ↑ | ↓ | N-↓ | |
| (a) Acute $CO_2$ loss | Hysterical and salicylate | ↑ | ↓ | N | Rebreathing and treating the cause restores levels |
| (b) Chronic $CO_2$ loss | Pulmonary fibrosis | ↑ | ↓ | ↓ | |

Johnston D.E. and Kaplan M.M. (1993) Pathogenesis and treatment of gallstones. *N. Engl. J. Med.*, **328**, 412–421.

# Renal stones (calculi)

There are four main types of renal calculi:
- 75% are calcium oxalate or calcium oxalate mixed with calcium phosphate and are associated with:
  (a) hypercalcaemia;
  (b) various causes of hypercalciuria without hypercalcaemia;
  (c) hyperuricosuria;
  (d) hyperoxaluria;
  (e) idiopathic.
- Triple stones (struvite) composed of magnesium ammonium phosphate usually associated with a previous infection by organisms with urea-splitting enzymes. This is the common mechanism for staghorn calculi.

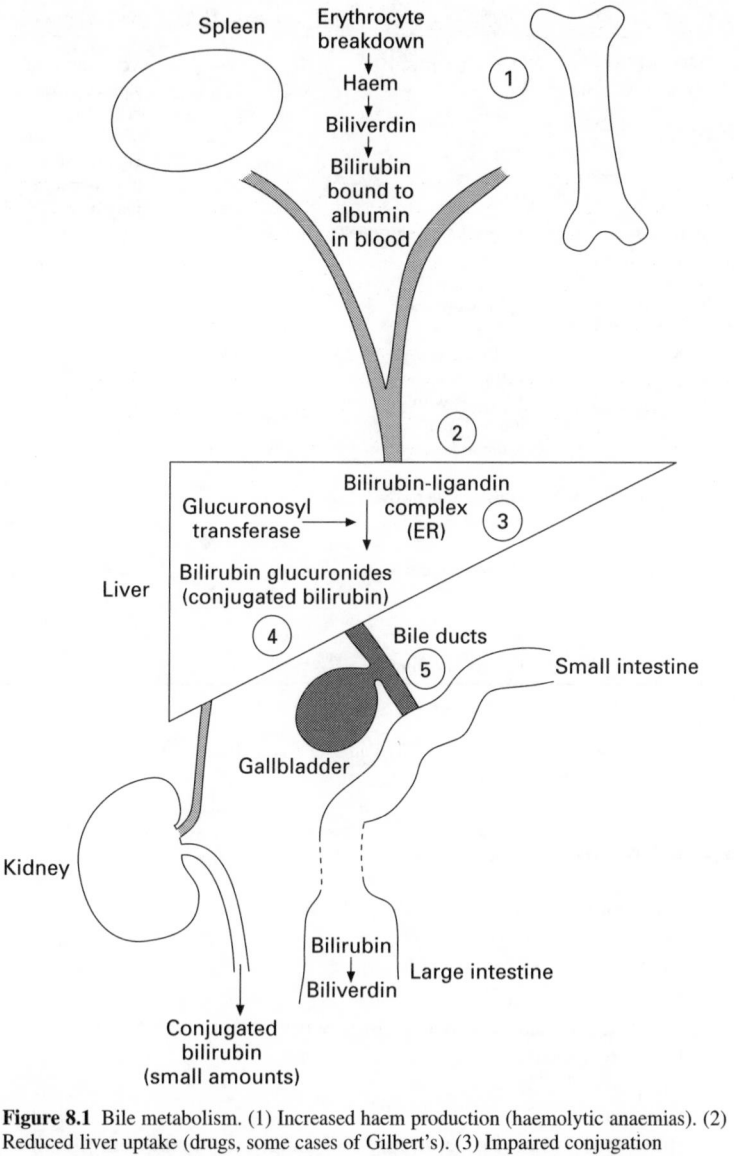

**Figure 8.1** Bile metabolism. (1) Increased haem production (haemolytic anaemias). (2) Reduced liver uptake (drugs, some cases of Gilbert's). (3) Impaired conjugation (physiological jaundice of newborn, Crigler–Najjar, most Gilbert's). (4) Impaired hepatic excretion (Dubin–Johnson, Rotor's, hepatocellular damage). (5) Intrahepatic and extrahepatic obstruction (stones, carcinoma, atresia, flukes)

- Uric acid stones are associated with gout and with diseases such as leukaemia with high rates of nucleic acid turnover.
- Cystine stones are associated with inherited disorders of metabolism of amino acids including cystine.

## Pathology

- All stones contain a mucopolysaccharide matrix but the most important determinant of stone formation is an increase in the urinary content of the materials that make up the stone.
- The precipitation of stones is also dependent upon pH, stasis, decrease in urinary volume and infection.
- Many stones occur in the absence of these factors and it may be that there are active factors preventing stone formation.
- Stones also predispose to infection and to eventual renal failure.
- Fragments of stones may break off and enter the ureters causing ureteric colic which is dramatically painful.

Coe F.L., Parks J.H. and Asplin J.R. (1992) The pathogenesis and treatment of kidney stones. *N. Engl. J. Med.*, **327**, 1141–1152.

# 9

# Haemodynamic disorders, ischaemia and shock

## Haemorrhage (loss of blood)

- Leakage from any part of the vascular system either internally or externally.
- Immediately following haemorrhage the indices of anaemia are normal and the pathological problems are caused by decreased volume.
- Over several hours fluid is diverted from its normal sites to correct the blood volume; blood indices now indicate an anaemia due to dilution.
- Following a mild haemorrhage the blood concentrations return to normal within a few days.
- Severe haemorrhage leads to shock and, if not corrected, can result in death. In severe haemorrhage the volume problems are complicated by the reduced gas-carrying capacity.
- Haemorrhage commonly results from vascular damage:
  (a) trauma;
  (b) atherosclerosis (aneurysms);
  (c) vasculitis;
  (d) erosion by neoplasms.

### Bleeding diatheses

Some patients have an increased tendency to bleed (bleeding diatheses) due to:
- vessel wall abnormalities:
  (a) infections;
  (b) inflammation;
  (c) scurvy;
  (d) hypersensitivity (drugs, Henoch–Schönlein purpura);
  (e) hereditary haemorrhagic telangiectasia.
- platelet disorders:
  (a) decreased production of platelets:
    (i)  bone marrow disease;

    (ii)  drugs, alcohol, virus.
  (b) decreased platelet survival:
    (i)  immunologic destruction;
    (ii)  disseminated intravascular coagulation (DIC);
    (iii) thrombotic thrombocytopenic purpura;
    (iv) vascular abnormalities (giant haemangioma).
  (c) sequestration in the spleen in hypersplenism;
  (d) abnormal platelet function:
    (i)  inborn errors of adhesion, aggregation or secretion;
    (ii)  drugs, i.e. aspirin.
- clotting factor abnormalities:
  - (a) haemophilias;
  - (b) liver failure.
- disseminated intravascular coagulation (DIC).

# Active and passive hyperaemia (accumulation of blood)

- Passive hyperaemia is also called congestion.
- Active hyperaemia is caused by vasodilatation to release heat as in exercise, fever and blushing.
- Passive hyperaemia is caused by local effects, such as impaired venous return, or systemic effects, such as heart failure.
- Passive hyperaemia is also usually associated with oedema.

# Haemostasis and thrombosis

- The blood is a liquid tissue contained in vessels of variable fragility so mechanisms exist for the solidification of blood to limit damage from trauma.
- When these mechanisms are activated to restrict the effects of trauma the process is called haemostasis.
- When they are activated inappropriately within the intact vascular system the end result is called thrombosis.

## Thrombosis

- Thrombosis is solidification of blood constituents within flowing blood in intact vessels in the living body.
- Clotting is solidification of the blood in static blood, or outside of a vessel, or outside of the body, or within a vessel in a dead body.

- This implies that thrombosis is an active pathological process and that clotting is a passive process.
- The appearance of clots and thrombi reflect this difference:
  - (a) thrombi are structured, often with alternating lines of platelets and blood constituents (lines of Zahn); clots settle in the plane of their container (vessel, corpse, test tube) with solid cellular components at the bottom ('redcurrent jelly') and solidified serum on the top ('chicken fat');
  - (b) thrombi are integrated clotting materials and are firm and elastic; clots are friable;
  - (c) thrombi are often adherent to the vascular damage that has caused them; clots are usually free in the vascular lumen or test tube.
- Thrombosis results from any stimulus that is sufficiently similar to the cues for haemostasis to trigger its mechanisms.
- There are three classes of mechanism that trigger thrombosis, traditionally referred to as Virchow's triad:
  - (a) changes in the vessel wall;
  - (b) changes in the blood flow;
  - (c) changes in the constitution of the blood (*Figure 9.1*).
- These three factors do not need to occur together to trigger thrombosis and some are more important in some situations than others.

### Fate of thrombi

- *Lysis*: the thrombolytic system may remove thrombi completely, especially small ones.
- *Organization*: the thrombus may become invaded by connective tissue elements and eventually be transformed into a scar; small ones may eventually become incorporated into the vessel wall.
- *Canalization*: following organization, new small vessels may grow through the thrombus eventually forming a single or numerous new channels.
- *Propagation*: because the thrombus itself slows blood flow it can cause further thrombosis and the clot may increase in length.
- *Clotting*: if a thrombus completely blocks a vessel and there is complete stasis, then simple clotting may occur; this is uncommon.
- *Embolization*: fragments of the thrombus may break off and move through the bloodstream until arrested in a vessel close to its own size causing occlusion of that vessel.

### Arterial thrombosis

- The commonest cause of arterial thrombosis is atherosclerosis.
- The vessels most commonly affected are the abdominal aorta, the

coronary, mesenteric, cerebral, renal and lower limb arteries.
- Atheroma is associated with relatively high pressure and only develops in the pulmonary arteries in pulmonary hypertension.
- Arterial thrombosis is most strongly associated with damage to vessel walls, while venous thrombosis is most associated with blood flow disturbances.
- Emboli are to distant arterial sites.

## Venous thrombosis

- The commonest cause of venous thrombosis is stasis.
- The main sites of venous thrombosis are calf veins and pelvic veins.
- Thrombi in the calf veins propagate into the iliac and femoral veins and emboli are generally from these.
- The structure of venous thrombi is much closer to that of blood clots due to the lower rate of blood flow in the veins.
- Emboli are to the lungs via the right side of the heart.

## Embolism

- Embolism is movement of solid, gaseous or imiscible material through the flowing bloodstream.

## Thromboembolism

- This is embolism of a thrombus.

### Arterial embolism

- Thrombi can embolize from arteries or veins.
- Thrombi embolizing from arteries (systemic embolism) deposit in arteries further along the arterial tree, towards the periphery of the tree.
- If they totally occlude such arteries, they produce relative ischaemia in the territory of supply.
- If there is no other supply to that area, it will die (infarction) and this is the most common sequel.
- If there is some collateral supply, the area may experience ischaemia but may survive at lowered functional level until the blockage is removed or until new vessels grow in to revascularize it.
- About 80% of systemic emboli come from the heart, these include:
  (a) emboli from myocardial infarction in the left ventricle (65%);
  (b) from vegetations on abnormal valves;
  (c) left atrial thrombi following atrial fibrillation.

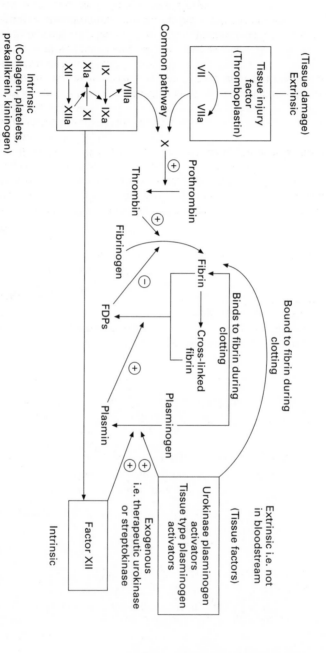

**Figure 9.1** Relationship of coagulation and fibrinolysis

## Venous embolism

- Venous thromboembolism gives rise to pulmonary embolism.
- These are classified into three grades depending on severity:
  - (a) small: these are often thrown off in showers and are unsymptomatic until their cumulative effect (often pulmonary fibrosis) begins to limit respiration;
  - (b) medium: these are symptomatic with dyspnoea, distress and chest pain. They also give physical signs such as respiratory/ventilatory mismatch and 'left strain' and ischaemic changes in $S_1Q_3T_3$ in the ECG;
  - (c) large: these present as sudden death.
- Heparin can be used to prevent the extension of thromboses, and streptokinase can be introduced onto the embolus via a long intravenous line

Bergqvist D. *et al* (1992) Prevention of venous thromboembolism after surgery: a review of enoxaparin. *Br. J. Surg.*, **79**, 495–498.

## Other causes of pulmonary embolism

- Amniotic fluid embolism (infusion):
  - (a) if the placental membranes tear and veins in the uterine wall or cervix are ruptured, either during delivery or in more rare causes of placental separation, then amniotic fluid consisting of squames, hair, fat mucin or bile may be 'injected' into the maternal circulation;
  - (b) this is a rare event (1 in 50 000) deliveries;
  - (c) with the disappearance of other causes of maternal death it is now the commonest cause;
  - (d) fatality from amniotic fluid embolism is about 85%;
  - (e) the mechanism of death is not dependent on emboli lodging in the circulation and blocking it; there is a poor correlation between severity of disease and volume of amniotic fluid in the lungs;
  - (f) it can be demonstrated with Atwood's stain (stains keratinocytes);
  - (g) it is thought that the effects are produced by thromboplastins in the amniotic fluid;
  - (h) death is due to uncontrollable DIC.
- Fat embolism:
  - (a) most commonly associated with long bone fractures (thought to be due to marrow fat release, but more probably due to metabolic processes in the blood);
  - (b) it also occurs in burns and soft tissue injury;
  - (c) it can be demonstrated in about 90% of multiple fracture cases;
  - (d) only 1% of multiple fracture cases develop the syndrome;
  - (e) symptoms develop 1–3 days after injury;

(f) symptoms consist of respiratory failure, neurological irritability proceeding to coma, thrombocytopenia causing petechial skin rash;

(g) it cannot be demonstrated in routine histology because fat is dissolved out in processing; frozen sections and fat stains such as oil red O are needed.

Hulman G. (1995) The pathogenesis of fat embolism. *J. Pathol.*, **176**, 3–9.

- Air embolism:
  (a) gases free within the bloodstream, i.e. not in solution, may act like any other emboli;
  (b) there are two main causes of air embolism:
    (i) gas entering the blood stream: gas (usually air) may enter the bloodstream from a number of causes:
      (1) injection (it needs 100 ml or more to cause problems);
      (2) neck trauma (including surgery); the low pressure cause air to flow in;
      (3) delivery or abortion; due to the pumping action of the contracting uterus;
      (4) pneumothorax (traumatic or surgical) with rupture of a large vein.

      The effects are frothy masses of gas and blood which act as occlusive emboli in the heart and lungs.
    (ii) gas dissolved in the blood coming out of solution: gas dissolved in the blood is usually related to breathing high-pressure gas mixtures during diving. Nitrogen dissolves and re-emerges as bubbles during rapid decompression. The acute form is the 'bends' or 'chokes'. The chronic form is caisson (from the French for 'box') disease. In the acute form the gas bubbles cause ischaemic pain by blocking small vessels in the musculoskeletal system (mostly around joints). The chronic form is caused by small foci of necrosis in these sites.
- Other emboli:
  (a) pieces of tumour may break off into the circulation and small fragments may enter the circulation more actively during metastasis;
  (b) atheromatous plaque may fragment and can settle anywhere, just as small arterial thromboemboli may do (cholesterol embolism);
  (c) foreign particles may be introduced if the ends of intravenous catheters break off during insertion;
  (d) infected thrombi from heart valves in bacterial endocarditis may break off to form mycotic aneurysms (in spite of the name these are usually bacterial not fungal).

## Ischaemia and infarction

- Infarction means 'stuffed full' and refers to situations in which there is blockage of blood flow out of a tissue but continued flow in, but it has come to mean death of the tissue in the living body due to vascular events.
- By definition infarction means death of tissue due to lack of oxygen and for practical purposes this is due to impaired blood supply.
- There are several descriptive terms for different infarcts based on colour and presence or absence of infection:
  (a) white infarcts are due to arterial occlusion in solid tissues such as heart, spleen and kidneys;
  (b) red infarcts are due to venous infarcts and occur in loose tissues (such as lung which also has a double circulation) or those with a double circulation or in those with previous congestion.
- Infarction caused by torsion is an example of infarction in the presence of congestion as the lower pressure venous system is occluded first and blood continues to flow in until the swelling stops all flow and infarction supervenes.
- Around the area of infarction there is often a zone of relative ischaemia and the breakdown products of tissue death may induce a reactive hyperaemia; this is well seen in the kidney where the infarct is a peripheral cone (seen as a triangle on section) representing the territory of the end artery which has been occluded and the periphery of this shows reactive hyperaemia.
- The end-result of most infarction is some form of fibrous scar.
- In the brain the infarcts usually result in a cystic area.
- Brain infarcts result from thrombosis, embolism or haemorrhage.
- Infarcts are also distinguished on the basis of infection and are termed septic or bland.
- Reperfusion injury: in many cases a restoration of perfusion worsens the damage. This is due to the existing damage which persists but is now supplied with oxygen which can be transformed into oxygen free radicals which themselves are very destructive. In experimental models this can be prevented to some extent by antioxidants.

Grace P.A. (1994) Ischaemia-reperfusion injury. *Br. J. Surg.*, **81**, 637–647.
Weller R.O. (1995) Subarachnoid haemorrhage and myths about saccular aneurysms. *J. Clin. Pathol.*, **48**, 1078–1081.
MacKenzie J.M. (1996) Intracerebral haemorrhage. *J. Clin. Pathol.*, **49**, 360–364.

## Hypertension

- Blood pressure persistently raised above the norm for the patient's age is termed hypertension.

- It is very common but difficult to set accurate criteria; in general a sustained diastolic above 90 mmHg or a sustained systolic above 140 mmHg is believed to carry an extra risk of complications.
- Hypertension is a major cause of morbidity and mortality in all Western-style communities.
- It is one of the most important risk factors in cerebrovascular accidents and in coronary heart disease as well as in congestive heart failure and renal failure.
- Over 90% of cases are idiopathic (essential hypertension).
- A small number of cases are secondary to other diseases:
  (a) renal disease due to high renin secretion;
  (b) increased intracranial pressure;
  (c) coarctation of the aorta;
  (d) vasculitis;
  (e) primary aldosteronism;
  (f) Cushing's syndrome;
  (g) phaeochromocytoma;
  (h) thyrotoxicosis;
  (i) oral contraceptives.
- Most hypertension is slow in development and the symptoms are insidious in onset (benign hypertension).
- Other less common forms are rapidly progressive and fatal at an early age (malignant hypertension).

## Pathogenesis of hypertension

- The manifestation of hypertension is raised blood pressure. This could be brought about by one of two basic mechanisms (or a combination of the two):
  (a) increase in cardiac output;
  (b) increase in vascular tone.
- Those who support the idea of primary increase in vessel tone suggest that the increased cardiac output is a response to this and that patients need their increased pressure to overcome the increased resistance.
- There is clinical support for this because elderly patients who have their hypertension aggressively returned to the levels typical of young individuals have many problems and may even suffer ischaemic events such as strokes.
- Those who believe that increased cardiac output is primary see the increased vascular tone as a physiological response to prevent overperfusion.

### Effects of benign hypertension

- It accelerates atheroma.
- It can cause hyaline arteriosclerosis; the effects are most marked in the kidney.
- Vascular rupture of Berry aneurysms may result, causing strokes.
- It can cause hypertensive retinopathy.

### Effects of malignant hypertension

- Effects are as for benign hypertension and hyperplastic arteriosclerosis with reduplication of arteriolar endothelium producing further narrowing of vessels (fibrinoid necrosis).

# Shock (circulatory collapse)

- Shock is a clinical situation resulting from an effective reduction in circulating volume and the body's responses.
- It may be caused by a true loss of blood volume or by expansion of the vascular capacity producing a relative diminution in circulating volume.
- The initial process may be complicated and obscured by the various physiological responses to the cause.

## Features of shock

### Primary effects

- Poor perfusion with eventual widespread anoxic tissue damage.
- Anoxic damage to endothelium causes more fluid loss due to leakage.
- Inadequate clearance of metabolites.
- Shift from aerobic to anaerobic metabolism with lactate accumulation and eventual lactic acidosis.

### Secondary effects (physiological responses)

- Adrenergic activation: peripheral vasoconstriction; sweating; increased pulse rate and cardiac output, antidiuretic hormone (ADH) secretion.
- Redistribution of perfusion, partly due to differing sensitivities to adrenergic drive.
- Lowered consciousness.

## Stages of shock

- Stages may be mixed, depending on the severity, or the patient may stay at one stage if the process is arrested.
- Three stages are usually described:
  (a) non-progressive;
  (b) progressive;
  (c) irreversible.

## Types of shock

- *Cardiogenic*:
  (a) pump failure due to: myocardial damage; dysrhythmias; tamponade; outflow obstruction (pulmonary embolus);
  (b) haemorrhagic (hypovolaemic);
  (c) loss of volume due to: bleeding; fluid loss from burns.
- *Septic*: severe bacteraemia from Gram-negative bacteria and less commonly from Gram-positive bacteria or fungi, caused by the production of severe peripheral vasodilatation.
- *Neurogenic*: anaesthetic accidents, spinal cord injury, products of conception wedged in the uterine os.
- *Anaphylactic*: due to generalized type I hypersensitivity reactions.

Barnett H.J., Eliasziw M. and Meldrum H.E. (1995) Drugs and surgery in the prevention of ischaemic strokes. *N. Engl. J. Med.,* **332,** 238–248.

Levin E.R. (1995) Endothelins. *N. Engl. J. Med.,* **333,** 356–363.

Weinmann E.E. and Salzman E.W. (1994) Deep-vein thrombosis. *N. Engl. J. Med.,* **331,** 1630–1641.

Parrillo J.E. (1993) Pathogenetic mechanisms of septic shock. *N. Engl. J. Med.,* **328,** 1471–1477

Welbourn C.R. and Young Y. (1992) Endotoxin, septic shock and acute lung injury: neutrophils, macrophages and inflammatory mediators. *Br. J. Surg.,* **79,** 998–1003.

Evans T.J. and Krausz T. (1994) Pathogenesis and pathology of shock. *Recent Adv. Histopathol.,* **16,** 21–47.

# 10

# Infections and surgery

## Abscess (*Table 10.1*)

- Defined as the accumulation of pus in a tissue space that eventually develops a 'pyogenic membrane' consisting of granulation tissue with polymorphs and fibroblasts.
- Subcutaneous abscesses, such as boils, 'point' and discharge onto the skin; if drainage is effective they leave only a small scar, but if they heal over still containing bacteria they may reform.
- Similarly the wall makes them very impenetrable for antibodies and antibiotics.
- Abscesses may also form within a hollow viscus, such as the gall-bladder, and may cause the natural drainage route to become obliterated by fibrosis, forming an empyema
- Such a sealed-off collection of pus may erode through the wall causing either a fistula or a sinus, depending on whether or not it connects with another hollow viscus.
- As it drains it may collapse and fibrose just as a subcutaneous abscess may.
- Cysts, which are enclosed spaces lined by epithelium, may become infected, attract polymorphs and the epithelium can be lost resulting in an abscess.

### Subcutaneous abscesses

- These may form from the introduction of bacteria via an injection site, or the bacteria may enter down an adnexal structure, commonly a hair follicle. Abscesses develop frequently in the axillae, groin and perineum (as in hidradenitis suppurativa).
- If they do not 'point' and discharge, they often need surgical drainage and may need to be held open with a wick, which is slowly withdrawn over some days or weeks allowing the cavity to granulate up and heal.

**Table 10.1 Causes of various abscesses**

| Site | Organisms | Comments |
|------|-----------|----------|
| Subcutaneous | *Staph. aureus* is by far the most common organism followed by *Strep. pyogenes* | Worldwide a great variety of organisms may be seen: *Bacteroides*; anaerobic cocci; and coliforms are often involved in abscesses around the anogenital region (anaerobes are often recognizable by the foul smell of the pus). *Mycobacteria*; *Pseudomonas*; *Nocardia*; and *Actinomyces* can be found in various parts of the world and in immigrants to the West |
| Cerebral | *Bacteroides fragilis* is usually from otogenic infection; sinus and haematologic spread from lungs tends to be *Strep. milleri*; surgical and accidental trauma may be associated with *Staph. aureus* | May be extradural, subdural or intracerebral, the organism depending on the source: *Bacteroides fragilis* often mixed with *E. coli*, *Proteus* or *Klebsiella*; *Strep. milleri* often mixed with respiratory organisms; cerebral abscess has declined in incidence but retains a mortality of 10–40% |
| Renal cortical abscess | Usually *Staph. aureus* | From haematogenous spread |
| Perinephric | Usually *Staph. aureus* | Commonly from rupture of renal cortical abscess |
| Lung | *Staph. aureus* or, rarely, *Klebsiella* infections may localize; *Bacteroides necrophorus* abscesses may occur behind obstructions; *Entamoeba histolytica* may be seen as an exotic import | Causes of lung abscess include: carcinoma; inhalation pneumonitis; inhaled foriegn body; infected cyst; infected pulmonary infarct; blood-borne secondary to staphylococcal septicaemia; secondary to lung infection. Drug addicts who develop influenza A are at increased risk of multiple lung abscesses containing *Staphylococcus* species |
| Liver | *Amoeba histolytica* (non-pyogenic) Pyogenic: non-sporing anaerobes (*Bacteroides fragilis*); coliforms (*E. coli*); *Strep. milleri* | *Amoeba histolytica* usually follows on chronic amoebic dysentary leading to amoebic hepatitis which may then localize as amoebic abscesses. Pyogenic liver abscess usually follows portal pyemia due to abdominal sepsis or infection of the biliary tract. Haematogenous spread from localized infection such as osteomyelitis may also occur |
| Peritonsillar | *Streptococcus* species | 'Quinsy' may develop from a streptococcal sore throat; much less common now |

# Wound infection

- In general a major determining factor in wound infection, however the wound is produced, is the state of the patient. High-risk patients include:
  - (e) elderly;
  - (b) debilitated (due to malignancy);
  - (c) malnourished;
  - (d) obese;
  - (e) diabetic
  - (f) infected;
  - (g) immunocompromised (due to malignancy, chemotherapy, steroids, acquired immuno deficiency syndrome (AIDS)).
- Any of these patients will have a higher postoperative wound infection risk and a higher tendency to infection following traumatic wounds.
- Traumatic wound infections (non-surgical wounds) are at risk of infection from the organisms in the environment in which the wound occurs and from the organisms carried by the patient in the tissues that are damaged.
- An added risk factor is the inclusion of foreign material in the wound or the presence of dead tissue.

## Surgical wound infections

Surgical wound infections are largely determined by the type of surgical wound and these are usually classified as:
- 'clean': this is surgery that does not penetrate the gastrointestinal tract, genitourinary tract or respiratory tract:
  - (a) infection rates are about 2–5%;
  - (b) the most common organism involved is *Staphylococcus aureus*;
  - (c) typical examples of 'clean' surgical operations are repairs of inguinal hernias or removal of subcutaneous lipomas.
- 'contaminated': any site of operation on tissue with a known normal flora (other than the skin) presents an increased risk of wound infection:
  - (a) the risk may be small when removing a non-inflamed appendix provided that spillage of bowel contents does not occur, but may be much increased if the appendix is gangrenous;
  - (b) wound infection risks are considerably raised in operations on the colon, mouth, gallbladder and vagina;
  - (c) the risks may reach 10–40%;
  - (d) pre-operative preparation by emptying the bowel or by antibiotic prophylaxis may reduce this risk in elective surgery;

(e) common organisms involved include *Bacteroides fragilis* and *Escherichia coli.*

- 'infected': the surgical site may be infected at the time of surgery, such as an abscess. Wound infection rates may approach 100% in these cases.

### Other factors affecting wound sepsis

- Prostheses (prosthetic hip joint or heart valve) or foreign bodies may encourage low-grade pathogens such as *Staphylococcus epidermidis.*
- The skill of the surgeon and general aseptic technique as well as the duration of operation all affect wound sepsis rates.
- The place of the operation in the list also affects rates; dirty operations should follow the clean ones.
- Highly contaminated carriers, particularly with active skin lesions, can increase *Staph. aureus* wound infection rates.
- Persistent structural abnormality, such as a leaking anastomosis, is a cause of wound infection as well as other problems.
- Patients who have been on the wards for several days prior to operation have a risk of developing new skin flora of more pathogenic strains.
- Good design of theatres and strict maintenance of standards of hygiene have greatly reduced the incidence of wound infection.
- Postoperative ward conditions also affect sepsis rates.

## Lower respiratory tract infection

A number of factors contribute to the development of lower respiratory tract infections in postsurgical patients:
- the debility following surgery;
- the general catabolic state of surgical patients;
- exposure to hospital pathogens;
- relative immunosuppression due to surgery;
- immobility for various reasons including strong analgesia and pain;
- shallow respiration due to postoperative pain.

## Septicaemia

- When bacteria are released into the blood there is a transient bacteraemia; if they begin to multiply in the blood and cause systemic symptoms this is septicaemia.
- Septicaemia may be present at emergency surgery, in which case the

nature of the organisms and their sensitivities may not be known and antibiotics must be given on a best-guess broad-spectrum basis.

- Even under emergency circumstances blood should be sent for culture and sensitivity before antibiotics are given in case those chosen prove not to be optimal.
- 'Contaminated' surgery is always at risk of producing septicaemia, as is any 'infected' surgery, and any pus from abscesses or other sites of infection should be sent for culture and sensitivity.

## Urinary tract infection

- Urinary tract infection is frequently a sign of anatomical abnormality (horseshoe or double kidney, duplex ureters, incompetent ureto-vesical valve) or calculi in the urinary tract and resulting in urinary reflux and ascending infection.
- It may also follow catheterization.
- Repeated episodes of infection may lead to acute pyelonephritis of one or both kidneys.
- The infecting organism is commonly *E. coli.*
- In some cases the whole kidney is replaced by pus (pyonephrosis).
- *Tuberculosis* may affect any or all of the urinary tract, commonly by haematogenous spread, and results in a sterile pyuria in which pus is seen but no organisms can be cultured by routine methods.
- The ureter may be thickened and the kidney may be completely destroyed and walled off as an enclosed mass of caseous and calcified material (autonephrectomy).

## Peritonitis

- Peritonitis can be a presenting symptom of an intra-abdominal catastrophe or a complication of surgery.
- It commonly results from a perforation of the gastrointestinal tract with leakage of irritant material (bile, pancreatic enzymes, gastric secretions) or bacterial-contaminated large bowel contents (*E. coli*, streptococci, *Staph. aureus*, Gram-negative rods and *Clostridium perfringens*).
- Peritonitis can also occur as a complication of septicaemia (pneumococcal, staphylococcal or streptococcal).
- Peritonitis from other infective causes produces inflammation of the viscera with consequent vasodilatation facilitating entry into the bloodstream and causing septicaemia.

- Another possible route is from the female genital tract following acute salpingitis or puerperal infection introducing gonococci and chlamydia.
- The infection may localize to produce subphrenic and subhepatic abscesses.
- Tuberculous peritonitis may also occur by spread from infected abdominal organs.

## Pyrexia of undetermined (unknown) origin (PUO)

- Infective causes are responsible for about three-quarters of acute cases but only one-third of chronic cases.
- This reflects the wide range of causes including:
  (a) infections (69% of acute, 36% of chronic);
  (b) neoplasms (6% of acute, 19% of chronic);
  (c) collagen diseases (3% of acute, 13% of chronic);
  (d) granulomatous disease;
  (e) endocrine disorders;
  (f) drug reactions;
  (g) central nervous system (CNS) disease;
  (h) tissue destruction;
  (i) transfusion reactions;
  (j) Munchausen's (and by proxy) syndrome.

## Opportunistic infections

Opportunistic infections are a disparate range of organisms with some features in common (*Table 10.2*):
- they are usually organisms of low pathogenicity;
- they are often commensals that only cause infections in the immuno-compromised individual;
- some may be conventional pathogens but when acting as opportunistic organisms may have unusual presentations;
- they include representatives of the viruses, fungi, bacteria, protozoa and metazoan parasites;
- opportunistic infections are a major cause of morbidity and mortality in immunosuppressed patients, AIDS, patients with malignancy and transplant patients;
- treatment must be based on accurate identification of the infective agent which necessitates a high degree of alertness in susceptible patients.

**Table 10.2 Opportunistic organisms (modified from Shanson, 1995)**

| Type of organism | Organism | Tissue | Comments |
|---|---|---|---|
| Bacteria | *Pseudomonas aeruginosa* *Klebsiella aerogenes* | Lung and blood | Gram-negative pneumonia, Gram-negative septicaemia |
| | *Staph. aureus* | Lung, blood, skin | Neutropenic patients; persistent and recurrent abscesses |
| | *Nocardia asteroides* | Lung, subcutaneous, kidney | Children with granulomatous disease |
| | BCG | Lung | Less common than tuberculosis in renal transplant patients but can affect children with granulomatous disease |
| | *Mycobacterium avium-intracellulare* | Disseminated | AIDS |
| Virus | Herpes simplex, cytommegalovirus, varicella/zoster | Can all cause fatal disseminated disease; simplex and varicella/zoster can cause severe skin, eye and mucocutaneous lesions | Lymphoma, immunosuppressed patients and AIDS |
| | Measles | Giant cell pneumonia | Leukaemic children and malnourished children |
| Fungus | *Candida albicans* | Bronchopulmonary, oesophageal, peritoneal, renal, blood, endocardium | Lymphoma/leukaemia, immunosuppression, AIDS |
| | *Cryptococcus neoformans* | Chronic granuloma in lung, CNS and disseminated | AIDS |
| | *Histoplasma capsulatum* | Pulmonary and disseminated | Organism endemic in N. America |
| Protozoa | *Pneumocystis carinii* | Interstitial pneumonia | AIDS |
| | *Toxoplasma gondii* | Brain, myocardium, disseminated | AIDS |
| | *Cryptosporidium* | Gastrointestinal tract | AIDS |
| Worm | *Strongyloides stercoralis* | Disseminated | May become disseminated long after it was acquired in endemic regions such as Guyana |

## Pseudomembranous colitis

- Many patients on antibiotics develop diarrhoea which usually subsides on withdrawal of the drug.
- Some patients develop a much more severe disease, characterized by fulminant colitis, profuse diarrhoea and dehydration leading, in extreme cases, to death.
- Pseudomembranes of fibrino-purulent necrotic inflammatory exudate develop and on histology these can be seen to be volcano-like eruptions of pus from the epithelial surface which are very characteristic.
- The process is due to the suppression of most of the bowel flora by the antibiotic except for *Clostidrium difficile* which overgrows.
- Occasionally the disease can develop with no history of antibiotic exposure following surgery.

## Helicobacter pylori

- Although it remains true that peptic ulceration is due to an imbalance between mucosal protective processes and the damaging properties of gastric acid and pepsin, the role of *Helicobacter pylori* appears to be central to most cases.
- This organism is present in 90–100% of patients with duodenal ulcer and in 70% of those with gastric ulcer.
- The mechanism of ulcer generation is believed to be due to bacterial urease producing ammonia and protease which breaks down glycoproteins in the protective gastric mucus.
- The underlying epithelial cells are exposed to acid and pepsin and the resulting inflamed area is digested, leading to ulcer formation.
- Elimination of *H. pylori* leads to ulcer healing and reinfection with the organism results in renewed gastritis, thus fulfilling Koch's postulates of infection.

# Implants

- Artificial implants such as mechanical heart valves or hip prostheses are prone to infection.
- *Streptococcus viridans* is the commonest cause of bacterial endocarditis both in patients who have had surgery and in those who have not.
- A wide variety of other organisms have been found in postsurgical cases:

(a) *Strep. faecalis*;
(b) *Staph aureus*;
(c) *Staph epidermidis*;
(d) diphtheroids;
(e) Gram-negative bacilli;
(f) fungi.

- Hip replacements may become infected at an early stage with resistant forms of *Staph. epidermidis*, which necessitates removal of the prosthesis.

Lucas S.B. (1989) Aspects of infectious disease. *Recent Adv. Histopathol.*, **14**, 281–302.

Millard P.R. and Esiri M.M. (1992) The pathology of AIDS: an update. *Recent Adv. Histopathol.*, **15**, 67–92.

Newell A. and Barton S.E. (1995) Testing healthcare staff for infection with HIV and hepatitis: logistic and ethical considerations. *J. Clin. Pathol.*, **48**, 885–889.

# Hepatitis B and C

- These are more of a risk for the surgeon than for the patient in a surgical setting.
- Infection can be acquired by needle-stick injury, as is the case with human immunodeficiency virus (HIV).
- Similarly the risk to patients from carriers of these viruses is a part of the risk of hospital-acquired infections.

Dhillon A.P. and Dusheiko D.M. (1995) Pathology of hepatitis C virus infection. *Histopathology*, **26**, 297–309.

Shanson D.C. (1995) *Microbiology in Clinical Practice*, 2nd edn. Butterworth-Heinemann.

# Disinfection/sterilization (modified from Shanson, 1995)

- Sterilization is the complete removal of all microbiological agents; disinfection is the reduction of potentially infectious agents to a level at which they are no longer capable of producing an infection.
- Sterilization can only be achieved on materials that are resistant to the sterilization process; it cannot be achieved with living tissues or patients – in these cases disinfection is the most that can be achieved.
- Many organisms have developed defence mechanisms against adverse conditions (such as spore formation) and this makes them difficult to kill by any means.

## Methods of disinfection

There are three main methods of disinfection:
- Cleaning: this means the removal of, commonly, biological materials from the object being disinfected. The most common form of cleaning is by washing (often with soap or detergent) and drying:
  - (a) this applies to hands, general equipment about the wards and theatres and floors, surfaces and cleaning implements;
  - (b) cleaning is often used in conjunction with other methods as a pretreatment to remove gross amounts of material that might provide some protection against heat or chemical disinfectants.
- Heating: the limitations of heating are the point at which the material being disinfected is itself adversely affected:
  - (a) low heat methods such as pasteurization heat material to 60°C for 30 min or 72°C for 20 s; these are called 'holder type process' and 'flash type process' respectively. It is the type of treatment that was developed for milk;
  - (b) to ensure efficient disinfection the devices used should have constant temperature monitoring and should automatically unlock only when the cycle is complete;
  - (c) devices that raise the temperature to 80°C for 1 min are recommended for bottles, bedpans, etc.;
  - (d) boiling raises the temperature to 100°C and kills most organisms, although some spores such as those of *Clostridium tetani* can resist boiling for long periods;
  - (e) the technique has considerable problems in practice and is seldom used now;
  - (f) autoclaves that reduce the atmospheric pressure allow water to boil at a lower temperature than 100°C so they can produce steam with equal disinfecting power but less destructive heat;
  - (g) the autoclaves operate automatically and provide disinfected, dry items at the end;
  - (h) some endoscopes may be treated in this way, particularly with the addition of formaldehyde to the system.
- Chemical methods: a variety of chemicals have been used for disinfection (*Table 10.3*):
  - (a) these include formaldehyde, glutaraldehyde, chlorine, iodine and ethylene oxide gas, most of which are toxic;
  - (b) chemical disinfectants which can be used on living tissues are called antiseptics.
- The efficiency of chemical disinfectants depends on many factors:
  - (a) the suitability of the disinfectant for the organism present;
  - (b) concentration;
  - (c) pH, temperature and volume of disinfectant;

**Table 10.3 Chemical disinfectants**

| Type of disinfectant | Specific disinfectant | Comments |
| --- | --- | --- |
| Alcohols | Isopropyl and ethyl | Kills most vegetative bacteria on smooth surfaces in 30 s. Not very effective against spores and fungi. Inflammable |
| Aldehydes | Glutaraldehyde and formaldehyde | Acts on spores, vegetative bacteria, viruses and fungi. Slow (exposure of 3 h for all bacteria to be killed). Not very effective against tuberculosis. Toxic and sensitizing. Glutaraldehyde needs to be fresh and alkaline |
| Diguanides | Chlorhexidine | Useful on skin against *Staph. aureus* |
| Halogens | Hypochlorites and chlorine | Active against spores, bacteria, viruses, fungi, hep B and HIV but easily inactivated by organic matter. Needs to be fresh. Iodophors and iodine are less active than hypochlorites and chlorine |
| Phenols | Phenol, chloroxylenol, soluble phenols (sudol and hycolin), hexachlorophene | Phenol is of historical interest. Fairly weak and narrow range |
| Quaternary ammonium compounds | Cetrimide and benzalkonium | Weak, used mostly in combination with chlorhexidine |

(d) inactivating agents such as large amounts of biological material not removed by prior cleaning;

(e) whether the disinfectant contains cultures of organisms resistant to it (often the case with mops and buckets used for 'cleaning' the ward).

## Methods of sterilization

There are three main methods of sterilization:
- heat:
  (a) dry heat:
      (i)   can be used in ovens on glassware, or for the destruction of biological waste by burning;
      (ii)  it is also used to sterilize the tips of forceps or inoculating wires and loops in the laboratory.
  (b) moist heat:
      (i)   is generated in autoclaves under increased pressure which allows the steam to reach temperatures greater than 100°C;

(ii) with steam sterilization the aim is to produce 'dry' steam which is highly penetrant; 'wet' steam contains water droplets and these prevent penetration;

(iii) most autoclaves have an automatic cycle and automatic temperature recording which indicate whether or not the cycle has been executed correctly;

(iv) it is usual to include material that indicates when the process has worked: bacteria are less commonly used these days but spore strips containing *Bacillus stearothermophilus* are included and are cultured for 5 days, negative culture indicating adequate sterilization of that load;

(v) Browne's tubes, which contain an indicator that changes from red to green when an adequate temperature has been maintained for long enough, are used twice a day to check adequate sterilization;

(vi) Bowie–Dick test measures the degree of penetration of the steam into the centre of a load with a St Andrew's cross that changes colour evenly across the whole tape when penetration is adequate.

- ionizing radiation can be used if dry or moist heat treatment is contra-indicated:
  (a) some plastic containers are discoloured or weakened by gamma rays;
  (b) high-speed electrons from a linear accelerator or cobalt-60 are used in practice and this makes the technique an industrial one rather than a hospital method of sterilization.
- ethylene oxide can be used for sterilization in the case of materials that are heat sensitive and is used industrially for prosthetic heart valves and plastic catheters:
  (a) the gas is toxic, inflammable and explosive and used at 60°C, so its use is restricted to industrial situations;
  (b) due to the necessity to eliminate all traces of the gas before the patient is exposed to the product it consequently is very slow.

## Hospital-acquired infection

- Hospital-acquired infection is also called nosocomial infection and may be exogenous or endogenous.
- Transmission from another patient in the hospital (cross-infection) or from the environment of the hospital (environmental infection) is exogenous.
- If the patient becomes infected from their own flora (self-infection), this is viewed as endogenous.

- Simple contact with infectious organisms seldom causes infection without the involvement of predisposing factors, as the organisms involved are those common in the general environment and which, if they cause any infection, cause much milder disease outside of the hospital.
- *Susceptibility* to infections is different in hospital patients since they are generally ill, immunosuppressed from disease or treatment or have had surgery which breeches normal barriers.
- *Contact* with other infected patients and the high density of people sharing the same facilities for cooking and ventilation, water supply and waste disposal all contribute to rapid rates of spread.
- *Staff* may have developed specialized and highly selected flora from long association with antibiotic-resistant strains due to selection and plasmid-mediated transfer of resistance.
- Some staff and patients may be natural carriers.
- *Non-human reservoirs* such as equipment and cleaning materials occur both in the ward and theatre environments.
- *Routes of transmission* include all of the usual routes (airborne droplets, skin scales, particles, direct contact with people and equipment) but in addition include surgical disruption of barriers, penetration of the vascular system and instrumentation such as catheters and drains.
- *Infection control* is the responsibility of good hospital management who should implement an *infection control policy* which should consist of two parts: the *infection control committee* and the *infection control team.*
- The control committee should meet regularly to formulate and update policy and the control team (usually headed by a medical microbiologist) should take day-to-day responsibility for implementation procedures.
- Factors controlled by the policy and the team should include:
  (a) sterilization procedures;
  (b) aseptic techniques;
  (c) cleaning and disinfection practice;
  (d) antisepsis procedures;
  (e) the use of antibiotics;
  (f) protective clothing;
  (g) isolation;
  (h) aspects of building and design;
  (i) storage and clinical use of equipment;
  (j) liaison with occupational health;
  (k) monitoring;
  (l) measurement of infection rates and hygiene standards.

# 11

# Ageing and death of the individual

- Ageing and death are closely associated.
- With progressive age death becomes more likely.
- The mechanistic view is that the older an object is the more likely it is that it will malfunction or totally cease to function.
- This is not a universal phenomenon; unicellular animals that reproduce by asexual division, in a sense live for ever. Amoeba alive today are in direct line of cytoplasmic and nuclear descent from the very first amoeba that ever lived.
- Single cells of multicellular animals do not behave like this, except for sperm and ova.
- Neurones and heart muscle cells become postmitotic around the time of birth and if one dies, it is not replaced.
- Even labile cells that can reproduce in the human body do so less efficiently with the passage of time.
- Older individuals show slower wound healing and they begin to show relative immune paresis.
- If cells from young animals are cultured they seem to be capable of about fifty cell divisions (Hayflick limit) but cells from older individuals are capable of progressively fewer cell divisions.
- Some individuals with a lower life expectancy also show a reduced Hayflick limit (Down's syndrome, progeria).

## Ageing

- Clinical features of old age.
- Arterial degeneration, particularly atherosclerosis, is one of the commonest causes of debility and death in developed countries.
- Many diseases may also have their origins in a progressively diminishing supply of oxygen and nutrients.
- In routine autopsies, however, it is not uncommon to see people who have apparently died of 'old age' without significant arterial disease.
- In many developing societies the aged population is not particularly afflicted by atherosclerosis and yet such individuals show all of the general signs of old age.

- It is very difficult in many cases to attribute death to any one disease state in the elderly.

## Theories of ageing

There are two main groups of ageing theories which are not necessarily mutually exclusive.

### *Inbuilt genetic mechanisms (clonal senescence theory)*

- Each animal species seems to have a characteristic natural life expectancy; not all individuals reach this under natural conditions prevailing in the wild.
- It may be that no individual reaches this natural limit because of the effects of predators, accidents and disease or the younger individuals may actively drive out or kill an aged member of the group or more passively neglect them when they are no longer useful or economically viable.
- If animals are kept under ideal conditions, it does appear that they age and die at around the same time. Barring accidents there is a characteristic lifespan.
- Most human cultures reflect this in their beliefs that there is a natural age at which to die (around 'three score years and ten', though modern estimates would put it around 75) and that there are natural phases in life: infancy, adolescence, adulthood and ageing.
- The processes of embryogenesis, infancy, adolescence and maturity are genetically programmed, although the individual experience of these stages in life may be very highly modified by environmental conditions; the current estimate is that the more complex and variable features such as behaviour are about 60% genetic and 40% environmental.
- The process of ageing seems to have a genetic component.
- Members of the same family tend to live to the same sort of age and age at the same sort of rate, leaving aside accident and disease; all animal species have recognizably characteristic lifespans, ranging from 1 day for a mayfly to well over 100 years for various amphibia.
- The actual inherited mechanism(s) that is responsible for the genetic component of ageing is still unclear but women generally live longer than men. Longevity appears to be inherited through the female line and all mammalian mitochondria come from the egg and none are transmitted via the sperm.
- Some gene(s) that have an effect on ageing are carried on chromosome 1 but the way in which they influence ageing is unclear.

- There are also some 'natural experiments' (progerias), genetic conditions such as Werner's syndrome, which show premature ageing and old age diseases such as advanced atheroma, whilst still chronologically in their teens or early adulthood.
- Down's syndrome patients generally age rapidly and it has been shown that their fibroblasts are capable of fewer cell divisions in culture than those from age-matched controls.
- These conditions may be true models of the ageing process in which the gene(s) for ageing is amplified or expressed early.
- Socio-economic correlations with ageing and death are more difficult to interpret; most diseases are more common in people from lower socio-economic groups and, given that people in these groups show ageing changes and die earlier than age- and sex-matched people from higher socio-economic groups, the most immediate interpretation is that people in these groups are disadvantaged in terms of diet, housing and social welfare generally and that this is the cause.
- However, a genetic interpretation could explain the data just as well.

### Wear and tear (replication senescence)

- This suggests that the normal loss of cells and the accumulation of sublethal damage in cells leads eventually to system failure.
- This theory provides a good explanation of why it is that cardiac and central nervous system failure are such common causes of death as the functionally important cells in these crucial tissues have no ability to regenerate.
- It depends upon a statistical view of ageing, suggesting that we are all exposed to roughly the same amount of wear and tear and therefore have a narrow range of life expectancy that appears to give us a characteristic lifespan.
- However, it is hard to reconcile this with the 1 day lifespan of the mayfly and its relatives (but of course humans *may* be unique).
- The various cellular and subcellular mechanisms that have been suggested as the cause of this sort of error accumulation include:
  (a) protein cross-linking;
  (b) DNA cross-linking;
  (c) true mutations in DNA making essential genes unavailable or functionally altered;
  (d) damage to mitochondria;
  (e) other defects in oxygen and nutrient utilization.
- The final common path may be the generation of 'free radicals'.
- The power of this theory lies in the mechanical analogy of wear and tear in machines but also in the way that it parallels our concepts of

the role of free radicals in some forms of carcinogenesis, particularly by those involving radiant energy.

- Living systems are distinguished from most mechanical systems by their ability to regenerate.
- However, the Hayflick phenomenon suggests that most cells have the capacity for only a limited number of divisions (unlike cancer cells which seem to be immortal) and that this is under genetic control.
- A possible mechanism of genetic control of ageing is telomerase.
- Telomerase is an enzyme that replaces sections of highly repetitive DNA located at the ends of chromosomes (telomeres).
- Telomeres are reduced in length by each successive cell replication cycle in somatic cells.
- Gametes (ova and sperm) have telomerase, as may malignant cells, which ensures their immortality.
- The telomeres have very few active genes and their mode of action is not known.
- In the final analysis *replicative* senescence seems to be dependent upon some form of *clonal* senescence and the modifications to the cell during its lifetime acts upon an intrinsic lifespan programme.

## Clinical features of ageing

- Chronological age of human subjects can often be estimated to within a decade or so on the basis of physical appearance, particularly in the elderly.
- There is some suggestion that ageing is a side-effect of development, proceeding from embryogenesis to maturity to old age.
- Maturity is the period of maximum reproductive capacity and is also the period of greatest prowess which permits the transmission of an individual's genetic characters.
- In old age the complex biological peak or prime begins to deteriorate and the chances of transmitting various genetic combinations decreases.
- The consequence of a cessation of reproductive capacity in the elderly is that diseases with a genetic component whose expression in a young adult might result in negative selection pressure has no such effect in the elderly and such diseases can therefore accumulate in the elderly forming the 'typical' diseases of old age.
- This obviously does not affect those genetic diseases which only become manifest in old age, as these individuals will already have reproduced and passed on the defective gene(s).
- Older individuals have had more opportunities for accidents (both gross and cellular) and the effect of this is that more show up in old age.

- The elderly will also be prone to accidents as a secondary function of failing eyesight, increased fragility of bones or decreasing mental acuity.

## Clinical appearances of ageing

### Ageing of skin

- Old skin is lax, wrinkled and repairs poorly.
- Skin on exposed areas is more affected than that on covered areas suggesting a relationship to sun exposure.
- Heavily sun-exposed skin is more affected than slightly exposed skin.
- Collagen gives tensile strength to the dermis; elastin provides elastic recoil.
- Sun (UV) exposure changes collagen and makes it weaker as well as causing a change in staining properties (it now stains with elastin stains = 'solar elastosis').
- True elastin is much reduced in quantity in elderly skin causing the laxness associated with old age.
- Collagen and elastin are both produced by fibroblasts but it is not known whether sunlight effects are on the proteins or the fibroblasts (the latter seems more likely).

### Osteoarticular ageing

- Osteopenia is the reduction of bone volume for any reason.
- Osteoporosis is a specific form of osteopenia associated with old age.
- Osteoporotic bone is much weaker than normal bone and may fracture spontaneously or from very minor trauma.
- Spontaneous collapse of vertebral bodies produces the common kyphosis of the elderly ('dowager's hump' clinically).
- The disease is much more common in postmenopausal women.
- Hormone replacement therapy (HRT) is protective.
- Other causes of osteoporosis include steroid hormones and malignant disease suggesting that hormonal and nutritional factors may play a role in the age-related form.
- Calcium supplements are largely ineffectual because it is the total amount of bone that is decreased – what is there is normally calcified.
- A significant factor seems to be that the amount of exercise and dietary vitamin D taken in youth is protective.

### Impaired immunity

- The efficiency of the immune system declines with age, not only with respect to new antigens but also to ones where the subject was immune previously.

- The increase in cancers in old age may be related to the decline in the activity of the immune system if immune surveillance for cancer is an effective mechanism of protection.
- Quiescent infections, such as tuberculosis and herpes zoster, may reactivate.
- Similar effects occur with therapeutic immunosuppression or that which accompanies malignancy.
- Paradoxically, there is also an increase in autoimmune disease with advancing age, suggesting that the prevention of autoimmunity is an active immunological process.
- However, this may be due to the fact that the elderly are more likely to have had some destructive disease of the organs (such as thyroiditis) that has released antigens and initiated an autoimmune reaction to them.

## Cardiovascular changes

- In Western-style societies death from cardiovascular disease is so common that it has come to be equated with death itself.
- Hypertension is another common association with the well-established causes of death.
- The basic cause of idiopathic hypertension is unknown, but it seems to begin with an increase in tone of small vessels and the increased blood pressure is a physiological attempt to push blood through the increased resistance, though the reverse is also possible.
- Unfortunately hypertension itself is damaging and is related to cardiovascular disease, strokes, retinopathy and renal failure.
- Although atheroma is associated with old age, the presumed precursor lesions (fatty streaks) can be recognized in very young adults.

## Fate of permanent cells

- Neurological function declines with age.
- Some of this may be due to blood vascular effects and to the development of the brain-specific amyloids of senile dementia but some is due to simple loss of neurones which cannot then be replaced.
- In the 'trade-off' between ageing and malignancy the neurones seem to have opted for ageing since their inability to replicate prevents them from neoplastic transformation (in the adult) but makes cell loss irreplaceable.

### Neoplastic diseases

- Some neoplasms are commoner in the young (such as retinoblastoma and neuroblastoma) but these are unusual tumours in many ways.
- Melanomas (except for lentigo maligna melanoma) are commoner in the young adult but these represent an unusual risk associated with lifestyle, as do cervical carcinomas.
- The usual pattern of neoplasia is that the incidence increases as a function of age.
- The development of neoplasia appears to be a statistical process and the elderly have had more opportunities.
- Some malignancies show a bimodal distribution, such as osteo-sarcoma which occurs in young adults and in the elderly.
- It is probable that these are two different tumours that are just morphologically indistinguishable; the ones developing in the elderly do so on the basis of chronic disease and regeneration, such as Paget's disease of bone or chronic osteomyelitis, those in young patients are of unknown aetiology.
- Many malignancies seem to arise on the basis of chronic damage and repair such as:
    - (a) Marjolin's squamous carcinoma in chronic ulceration of the lower limb;
    - (b) hepatocellular carcinoma in alcohol abuse;
    - (c) carcinoma of the lung in smokers;
    - (d) mesothelioma in asbestos exposure.

# Death

- The United Nations statistic defines death as the permanent disappearance of all signs of life.
- Living systems are able to maintain homeostasis in the presence of fluctuations in the environment, dead ones cannot.
- The processes that lead to death in some way disrupt homeostatic mechanisms.
- Clinically this is often seen as:
    - (a) overwhelming trauma;
    - (b) overwhelming sepsis;
    - (c) overwhelming shock;
    - (d) overwhelming disease of a vital organ;
    - (e) inability to halt a progressive disease state.

## Dying and death

- These are distinct phenomena, although the *process* of dying often precedes the *event* of death.
- A person killed in a sudden accident was not necessarily dying up until that point.
- A person who is dying from shock or haemorrhage does not have to die if effective treatment is instigated.

## Clinical features of death

- The determination of death depends upon the absence of 'vital signs':
  (a) respiration (both by observation and aided by the stethoscope);
  (b) pulses (at the wrist, in the neck, in the groins);
  (c) responses to progressively deeper pain;
  (d) stagnation in the circulation in the form of 'beading' of blood in the arteries (can be seen in the retina).
- The absence of these signs is difficult to demonstrate in some cases, particularly in:
  (a) hypothermia;
  (b) neurological coma;
  (c) drowning;
  (d) drug overdose;
  (e) endocrine causes of coma.
- In the absence of contraindications, cardiopulmonary resuscitation may be attempted.
- If the patient is unrousable, then in the hospital situation the tests may be performed again after a delay.
- The need to determine death with accuracy and rapidity has been highlighted by the needs of organ donation and rules have been established for this:
  (a) the pupils are fixed in diameter and do not respond to sharp changes in the intensity of incident light;
  (b) there is no corneal reflex;
  (c) the vestibulo-ocular reflexes are absent;
  (d) no motor responses within the cranial nerve distribution can be elicited by adequate stimulation of any somatic area;
  (e) there is no gag reflex or reflex response to bronchial stimulation by a suction catheter passed down the trachea;
  (f) no respiratory movements occur when the patient is disconnected from the mechanical ventilator for long enough to ensure that the arterial $CO_2$ level rises above the threshold for stimulation of respiration.

- It is important to recognize that factors such as body temperature and the presence of drugs can modify this.
- The application of these tests is restricted to experts with a suitable level of expertise, in the presence of another, independent doctor who must not be part of the transplant team.

Cotton D.W.K. (1995) Death; the individual. *Prog. Pathol.*, **1**, 1–11.

## Sudden infant death syndrome

- This category of deaths, together with the less well known adult variant, remains obscure by definition.
- It occurs in young children, is associated with a wide range of social childcare habits and its causation remains obscure.
- It may be a collection of disparate and, as yet, unrecognized disease states, possibly related to the infant's social condition or it is still possible that it is an aberrant early expression of a 'death gene'.
- The term 'sudden infant death syndrome' is used only when an exhaustive post-mortem examination fails to reveal an identifiable cause of death.

## The Coroner

- This is an ancient office set up to determine causes of death in the community and to provide regulation of unlawful causes of death.
- The coronial system operates in most countries where there is a history of British influence; countries with a history of the Code Napoleon have a different system and Scotland operates an office called the Procurator Fiscal.
- In some states in the USA the role of coroner and forensic pathologist has been fused to produce an office called the Medical Examiner.
- In England and Wales coroners may be legally qualified or medically qualified or, in some jurisdictions, both.
- They are assisted by coroner's officers who are generally, but not necessarily, police officers.
- There is a common law duty on all individuals to report suspicious deaths to the coroner but the majority of cases are reported by doctors and police officers.
- The coroner may require an autopsy and may hold an inquest but it is his decision and neither can be refused.
- The coroner has the duty to investigate certain classes of deaths:
  (a) deaths in which the body is unidentified;

(b) if the certifying doctor is not certain of the cause of death;

(c) when there is any suggestion of suspicious circumstances or history of violence (including murder and suicide);

(d) deaths as a result of an accident (there is no time limit);

(e) death due to industrial disease or work related;

(f) deaths linked with abortions;

(g) deaths during surgery or before full recovery from an anaesthetic (or related to anaesthesia or any other medical procedure or investigation);

(h) where the actions of the deceased may have contributed to death (self-neglect, drug abuse);

(i) if the death occurred in police or prison custody;

(j) if the deceased was in receipt of an Armed Forces pension.

- There are two other situations where reporting is not a statutory requirement but is recommended local practice in most jurisdictions:

  (a) deaths occurring within 24 h of admission to hospital;

  (b) where the deceased was detained under the Mental Health Act.

## Autopsies

- The terms autopsy, necropsy and post-mortem are used interchangeably.
- The most accurate is probably 'necropsy' but the term in most common use is 'autopsy'.
- If the coroner determines that a hospital death does not fall within his jurisdiction, then it is legitimate to ask the relatives for permission to perform an autopsy ('request', 'consent' or 'hospital' autopsy).
- Consent must be informed and the relatives have absolute rights of refusal in whole or part.
- If they refuse it is improper to then seek a coroner's autopsy, as this should have preference anyway.
- Relatives have no right to refuse a coroner's autopsy because, in suspicious cases, this would be open to abuse.
- Material from the autopsy may be retained for research or teaching in a hospital autopsy, but not in a coroner's autopsy unless it is relevant to determining the cause of death.
- In consent autopsies the technique can be modified to a limited autopsy with not all cavities opened or not all organs examined.
- In extreme cases (some infection cases) the autopsy can be restricted to sampling of tissues by needle autopsy (using Tru-cut needles).
- The rate of hospital autopsies is falling steadily.
- The utility of autopsies is shown by the fact that much health care planning is based on death certification and it has been shown

many times that the rate of disagreement between causes of death recorded before autopsy compared to the findings at autopsy is very high (15–30%), even in cases where clinical confidence was very high.

Start R.D. and Cotton D.W.K. (1995) Autopsies and the surgeon. *Surgery*, **13**, 239–240.
Start R.D. and Cotton D.W.K. (1996) The current status of the autopsy. *Prog. Pathol.*, **3**, 179–188.

# Index